The 21ˢᵀ Century Diet

THE 21ST CENTURY DIET

Lynne Waller Scanlon

ST. MARTIN'S PRESS   New York

Design by Stanley S. Drate/Folio Graphics Co. Inc.

Library of Congress Cataloging in Publication Data

Scanlon, Lynne Waller.
     The 21st century diet.

     Includes index.
     1. Reducing diets.   2. Biological rhythms.   I. Title.
II. Title: Twenty-first century diet.
RM222.2.S254   1984   613.2'5   83-24662
ISBN 0-312-82421-1

First Edition
10 9 8 7 6 5 4 3 2 1

To my family and friends, all of whom have been incredibly supportive and encouraging during all phases of this book and my previous books.

To Ron Green and Joe McAlonen for their kindness and generosity.

CONTENTS

7

The 25 + Pound Problem 71

Compulsive Overeating . . . The Alcoholism Connection . . . Questionnaire: Are You Addicted to Food? . . . Breaking Food Addiction . . . Eleven People Who Can Help You . . . The Food Elimination Method . . . The Rinkle Mono-Diet Method . . . The Food Abstention Method

8

Taking the Obsession out of Dieting 89

Calories: Avoid 'em, Burn 'em, and Reinforce Their Departure . . . Are Your Personal Goals Sufficient Motivation? . . . Losing Weight to Improve Health . . . Losing Weight to Look More Attractive . . . Losing Weight to Be More Agile . . . The Secret to Making the 21st Century Diet Your Last Diet Effort . . . Why You Keep Losing the Same Old Pounds . . . Option #1—Reducing Your Energy Crisis . . . Option #2—Gentle Group Pressure and Encouragement . . . Option #3—The Tripartite Approach . . . The Best Time of Day to Exercise . . .Exercise? *Moi?*

9

Pre-Diet Questions and Answers 104

Meal Substitutions? . . . Allergies? . . . Dining Out? . . . Diet Pills? . . . Not a Breakfast Eater? . . . Exercise? . . . Alcohol? . . . Time to Begin? . . . Hints Prior to Beginning?

13

Slim and Trim Forever?   171

You Already Have What It Takes . . . Approximate
Calories Needed to Maintain Weight Levels . . .
Sorting Through Governmental and Institutional
Dietary Recommendations . . . The Reverse Pyramid
Food Guide . . . The 4-Day Food Rotation Guide
. . . Watch Out for Holiday Calories . . . Watch Out
for Subtle "Natural Changes" That Influence Weight
Control . . . Begin or Keep Exercising . . . Eat "Close
to Natural" Foods . . . The 21st Century Diet

Appendix   187

Food Families • Protein and Caloric Content of
Cheeses • Fruit and Vegetable Drink Calories

Index   207

Acknowledgments

The Doctors and the Scientists

Theron Randolph, M.D., is a physician whose pioneering work led to discoveries about food allergy and a phenomenon called "food addiction." Portions of his findings are integrated into *The 21st Century Diet*.

Charles F. Ehret, Ph.D., senior scientist at the Argonne National Laboratory, has devoted his professional life to the study of daily or "circadian" rhythms. The information he has discovered relating to how and why man responds, biochemically, to food has been incorporated into the overall program of *The 21st Century Diet*.

Herbert Rinkle, M.D., originator of the Rinkle Mono-Diet and the Rotary Diversified Diet, and a physician considered one of the greatest clinicians in the field of bioecologic illness, has developed invaluable techniques for isolating the overweight person's problem foods. His extraordinary contributions to the medical and scientific community and his techniques to eliminate "food addiction" have helped thousands of people. His work is also included in *The 21st Century Diet*.

Roger J. Williams, Ph.D., former president of the American Chemical Society, now director of the Clayton Foundation Biochemical Institute at the University of Texas, and discoverer of pantothenic acid, has developed a vitamin and mineral formula that takes the guesswork out of dietary supplements. His suggested daily supplement is included, as well, in *The 21st Century Diet*.

Incorporated into *The 21st Century Diet* is information from the above researchers, along with that from hundreds of their fellow physicians, professors, and scientists as published in professional journals including *The American Journal of Medicine, The Journal of Dietary Nutrition, The Journal of Nutrition, Public Health Reports, Journal of Food Science, American Dietetic Association Journal, Nutrition Today, Journal of the American Medical Association, Psychosomatic Medicine, Journal of Nutrition Education, American Journal of Clinical Nutrition, Addictive Behavior, International Journal of Obesity, New England Journal of Medicine, Post Graduate Medicine, The Ecologist Quarterly.*

With thousands of documented case histories among them, these brilliant men and women have broken new ground in areas of research that offer hope, at last, to countless overweight men, women, and children.

FOREWORD

About seven years ago, as a health and science writer, I initiated a project that was to result in a best-selling book, *Dr. Mandell's 5-Day Allergy Relief System*. More through happenstance than anything else, I stumbled across information that to me—and eventually to the hundreds of thousands of people who bought the book—seemed so exciting, so vital, so worthy of widespread dissemination, that I suggested to my eventual co-author, Marshall Mandell, that he and I work on a book project together. While researching the book, I realized that Dr. Mandell was a disciple of Theron Randolph, M.D., a physician who pioneered investigation into a field of medicine that would eventually be called *bioecology*. As the premier researcher in the area of bioecology, Dr. Randolph had discovered a link between food allergy and obesity. It was he who first demonstrated clearly that there exists an "addictive" form of food allergy, and that this dependency on certain foods can be broken. What wonderful news for those men, women, and children who fight an endless battle with weight! It isn't caused by lack of will power, or oral fixation, or poor eating habits. No! The problem often has its origins in illness—the illness of addictive food allergy.

As I finished writing *Dr. Mandell's 5-Day Allergy Relief System*, I made a mental note to pursue this fascinating topic in depth at a later date.

My next project was with Charles F. Ehret, Ph.D., senior scientist at the Argonne National Laboratory outside Chicago, Illinois. Dr. Ehret is one of the most eminent scientists in the field of chrono-biology (biological rhythms), a researcher who works closely with

NASA, NATO, the airlines, and major corporations to understand the human body's natural rhythms. During the course of my research for *Overcoming Jet Lag*, a book designed to aid the long-distance traveler suffering from disrupted body rhythms, more information related to diet and health began to surface. Human body rhythms, it turns out, have cycles that are split-second, daily, weekly, and yearly—and some cycles affect weight gain and loss, the efficiency of metabolism, and the urge to eat on not only a daily but also on a seasonal basis.

Again, I thought, this information definitely pertained to people on diets, too. If I were to combine this with the information I had obtained during the research for my previous book . . .

Suddenly, a file I had labeled "potential diet book" began to fill up with clips from articles from a variety of sources. Some came from popular magazines (and gave me leads to follow up on), but most I discovered here and there among the stacks of scientific journals that I invariably have to scour in the pursuit of relevant data for whatever project I am working on at the time.

As I continued to accumulate findings from a variety of scientific researchers who were diligently working in their own particular fields, I began to realize that bits and pieces of seemingly unconnected discoveries actually were all interrelated and had real significance for dieters. Although the researchers were all brilliant scientists, so specialized were their areas of experience and interest that only an outside observer seeking data that pertained to weight loss would notice that these discoveries had great worth for dieters. Not being particularly devoted to any one scientific pursuit—chronobiology or bioecology, for example—I was able to branch out and investigate research from any and all fields.

What I pieced together was extremely exciting. By pursuing information from myriad fields, I realized that a bold new approach to dieting could be developed. By putting all these seemingly disparate facts together, I began to evolve a systematic approach.

As an occasional dieter myself, I was particularly interested in how to go about dieting *once*—and make that once enough. Surely, I thought, there must be a solution to keeping weight under control forever, without constant monitoring. I did not mind the thought of making one big effort to get down to the proper weight, but what I did detest was having to make that effort over and over. Once should be enough! With *The 21st Century Diet*, I believe you will find it is.

LYNNE WALLER SCANLON

The 21st Century Diet

1

Introducing:
The 21ˢᵀ Century Diet

FACT: You are about to participate in a boldly different kind of weight reduction and maintenance plan.

FACT: You will receive *new* information that was until now unavailable from the scientific and medical community.

FACT: You will understand for the first time what has really caused your weight gain and can master *proven* methods to reverse it.

FACT: You can make The 21st Century Diet your *last* diet ever!

A Diet for the 21st Century

A diet for the 21st century? Yes! At last there is a medically sound diet that combines 20th-century advances in science and medicine from hospitals and laboratories throughout the world into an approach designed for the 21st century. Indeed, *The 21st Century Diet* takes the conclusions drawn by esteemed researchers from a variety of fields in science and medicine and synthesizes those discoveries that relate directly to diet and dieting into an entirely new concept. Exciting and innovative, *The 21st Century Diet* presents new information and a unique plan that virtually assures the dieter successful weight reduction—and successful weight maintenance. So new is the information contained in *The 21st Century Diet* that even the vast majority of physicians, nutritionists, and health groups, not to mention dieters, are unaware of its vital significance.

1

The Knowledge You Need to Succeed

The mechanism of weight gain and loss is no mystery, particularly to those inveterate dieters with three wardrobes—small, medium, and large—hanging in their closets. Scientists have long known that weight gain is simply the result of the number of the calories consumed exceeding the number of calories expended. Weight loss occurs when you either eat fewer calories, burn off more calories, or combine both. What has remained a mystery, however, is why once you take the weight off you cannot, despite your best intentions, keep it off. Half the people in America have dieted at least once in the last five years, and one out of four of those same dieters has dieted *five times* or more over that five-year period![1] The same pounds keep disappearing and then reappearing, often as quickly as they take them off. It is entirely possible that over the course of a lifetime, if every year you gain and take off the same sixteen pounds,[2] you could have shed 800 pounds! This may sound like a great deal of weight, and it is, but it is nothing compared to the types of statistics that would apply if you are one of the people who diet as frequently as the seasons change.

What is the problem? Why the continual necessity to diet and rediet? How can you make The 21st Century Diet your last diet? Within *The 21st Century Diet* you will find information that answers your questions about dieting, including why dieting to reach your desired weight is so difficult, and why, if you do manage to lose weight, it seems nearly impossible to keep it off. *The 21st Century Diet* includes, as well, information that explains

- why it is more difficult (but not impossible) to diet during specific months of the year because of *prehistoric instincts* and *circadian rhythms;*
- why the typical dieter's high carbohydrate breakfast of toast, fruit, and/or coffee is the *worst* possible breakfast a dieter can have if he or she wants both appetite suppression and energy;
- why it is best to rotate your foods and try not to eat the same food more frequently than once every four days;
- why predominantly high-protein meals should be eaten only at certain times of the day;

- why the *addictive* aspect of foods exists as a *food allergy,* and how to break food addiction within four days, forever;
- why depending on your size and activity levels, at least 800, 1200, or 1600 calories must be consumed each day in order for you to satisfy your metabolic needs, diet successfully, and stave off hunger pangs;
- why diet pills fail even though they eliminate appetite;
- why coffee and tea actually *produce* fatigue in the morning, and tend to make your diet plan more difficult;
- why timing and composition of meals are as important to the diet as the number of calories consumed—how dieters who consumed 2000 calories in the daytime lost weight and dieters who consumed 2000 calories during the evening gained weight;
- why changes of lifestyle (job, marriage, college, retirement, etc.) can result in the need to diet, yet other lifestyle changes (temporary injury, illness, etc.) do not necessarily do so;
- why supplements are vital in today's world of vitamin- and mineral-depleted foods if you are to be truly healthy.

Indeed, The 21st Century Diet provides an amazingly easy, completely sound, and tremendously rational approach to weight loss. With information gathered from personal interviews with scientific authorities, supplemented by independent research reported in the most highly respected professional and medical journals, *The 21st Century Diet* arms the dieter with the kind of information needed to conquer weight gain, not just temporarily reverse it. Ultimately, *The 21st Century Diet* offers the dieter all the knowledge needed to understand why weight has become a problem and what it will take to remedy the situation once and forever.

Is the diet practical? Absolutely. The 21st Century Diet can be easily incorporated into your daily routine, whether you have a great deal of free time or practically none at all, whether you are eating at home or dining out. Is it quick? Yes. The program allows for initial dramatic weight loss while still providing for sustained weight loss. Is it healthy? Definitely. Because it is derived from the latest data available, The 21st Century Diet is based on facts, not magical premises, and provides the opportunity for optimum weight loss by creating optimal diet conditions.

The *Three* Plans of the 21st Century Diet

There are three special weight reduction plans from which a dieter can choose on The 21st Century Diet:

The 800-Calorie Plan—ideal for very short and/or very sedentary dieters.

The 1200-Calorie Plan—ideal for average height and/or moderately active dieters.

The 1600-Calorie Plan—ideal for tall, extremely active and/or extraordinarily overweight dieters.

Why THREE plans? Since your particular body frame may be either small, medium, or large or a combination of frames (small from the waist up, large below, for example, as explained later), each plan on The 21st Century Diet is especially designed for men and women who share what has proved to be the most significant characteristics when it comes to dieting, such as height, activity level, and amount of weight loss being sought.

The Height Factor: A "calorie" is not a "thing," but a unit of the "energy" your body needs to grow, repair itself, and function in general. Through a process called "metabolism," energy is extracted either from incoming food or, when the amount of incoming food is not sufficient to meet your energy requirements, from stored reserves. Of all the calories you actually use each day (an amount that varies depending upon how active your day is), a minimum amount is necessary to keep your heart beating, lungs pumping, and temperature normal, even if you are just lying in bed and barely moving. This is known as your resting or basal metabolism rate. In addition, since a shorter person with less mass to sustain requires fewer calories per day than a taller person to meet minimum caloric needs, height is one of the major factors you should take into account when deciding upon the diet plan for you.

Activity Levels: The amount of physical activity in your daily life is another important factor. If a walk to the mailbox at the end of the driveway is about as much activity as you get, your caloric needs (beyond those of your basal metabolic needs, which are separate) are far fewer than if you were more active, or even an athlete. Physical activity "burns" calories, and if you are moderately or extremely active during the course of a day, you can require and should allow yourself a few hundred extra calories as your minimum. After all, you will not only be cutting down on food intake, but simultaneously burning those calories you do allow yourself. Although you may be eating foods containing 1200 or 1600 calories per day, by taking into account the hundreds you burn off during your physical activities you can end up by actually allowing several hundred calories *fewer* into your system.

The Weight Factor: The third aspect is an important one, too. If you are between 25 and 100+ pounds overweight, there is absolutely no need to limit yourself to 800 or even 1200 calories per day until you shed a great deal of weight. The 1600-calorie diet will represent such a decrease in caloric intake that you will see dramatic results without shocking your system by sudden, extreme calorie deprivation. In addition, people with extremely large amounts of weight to lose, or those people who cannot seem to lose weight no matter how severely they diet, will find, as explained in detail later, that they stabilize their systems with The 21st Century Diet, and can finally begin to lose weight.

Getting Started

Your first step in The 21st Century Diet should be to read all the information contained in this book, cover to cover, to get an overview of the types of approaches that are involved and to help determine the categories into which you may fall. Your second step should be to choose from one of the three plans offered: the 800-Calorie Plan, the 1200-Calorie Plan, or the 1600-Calorie Plan, whichever is appropriate for your height, activity level, or weight. Your third step should be to go on to formulate your own "customized" 21st Century Diet, based upon the information gleaned from the pages of this book, and from the experience you will gain in actually dieting successfully and enjoyably.

NOTES

1. Earl Ubell, "Health on Parade," *Parade Magazine,* 13 February 1983, p. 13.
2. The average number of pounds lost during a diet. Ibid., p. 14.

2

A High-Tech Being in a Stone-Age Body

FACT: You instinctively prefer sweet-tasting foods.

FACT: You eat meat to excess because of prehistoric instincts.

FACT: You have more trouble dieting during the winter because of an instinctive mechanism that anticipates months of hardship.

An Objective Look at Today's Homo Sapiens

One of the reasons dieting can be so difficult is because you have to resist your own instincts in order to succeed. While it might sound far-fetched to suggest that a species as highly evolved as mankind is influenced by traits developed in prehistoric times, it is true. Even though they often seem dormant, mankind's instincts are as immutable and formidable as they were millions of years ago. They are a natural and inborn mode of response that has, as part of man's adaptive process, become hereditary and imbedded in the genes of the human being. Even though millions of years and millions of generations have passed since the dawn of man, instincts remain as much a part of us as we are a part of the earth. Developed as a result of mankind's adaptive process, instincts are directly responsible for man's survival as a species while other animals suffered extinction. So essential were instincts to survival that even today they continue to exert a tremendous influence over man's actions. The "flee or flight" instinct, for example, surfaces during times of potential violence or hazard during which you weigh the opportunity for successful retaliation against the advisability of a quick departure. The reproductive instinct assures the propagation of the species. The sucking instinct of newborns enables them to know how to nurse immediately after birth. No less strong are the instincts that come into play when you attempt to diet.

Our minds may have entered the age of high technology, but our bodies have hardly graduated from the stone age. Human beings can put astronauts on the moon and investigate the black holes of space, but when it comes to genetic programming, man remains essentially the same being that he was millions of years ago, when he and his fellow beings populated the forests and savannas and foraged for food, relying on wiles and instinct to survive. His choice of food was selected from among substances also eaten by other living creatures, though that choice was based on such factors as what he could acquire with his limited physical prowess, what he could chew easily with his particular type of "differentiated" tooth arrangement, and what he could digest in his stomach. His selection was also affected by seasonal changes and availability. For the most part he relied on a huge variety of plants to sustain him, and occasionally, very occasionally, a piece of meat to supplement his essentially vegetarian diet.

THE INSTINCTIVE EATING OF SWEETS

It didn't take highly evolved intelligence for early man to realize that not only was he vulnerable to predators, the elements, and other humans, but he was also surrounded by vegetation from which he would have to make constant selections as a means of survival. From among the vegetation available to him, man learned, by trial and error, that those items that were sweet tasting were not lethal, while those items that were bitter or sour occasionally had the capacity to make him very ill or even kill him. If something tasted sweet and did not hurt him, but something sour had the potential to do him great harm, elementary reasoning caused him to shy away from the latter. During the course of millions of years, the safety factor inherent in a food that was sweet caused man to develop a "sweet tooth" as an instinctive tool of survival.

Even when tiny babies, who have never been exposed to anything other than mother's milk, are fed something sweet, like honey, they immediately show by facial expressions a decided preference for the sweet food over something nonsweet.[1] Like their ancestors before them, children instinctively reject something tart or sour. Even as they grow older and learn intellectually that sugar causes cavities, and a cavity necessitates a trip to the dreaded dentist, children still clamor for sweets. Adults, grown children that they are, also respond to this instinctive preference for sweet food.

When naturally sweet fruit (or honey) was available, early man ate it and enjoyed it, but the staples of his diet came from among the various grasses, nuts, leaves, stalks, and the like that were available to him. Today, however, sweet-tasting food is everywhere, and by no means limited to *fructose*, the sugar found in sweet fruits and honey. Although mankind still has naturally sweet foods from which to choose, he also has an abundance of items that have been artificially sweetened through the use of *sucrose*, the sugar extracted and refined from sugarcane or sugar beets. Cakes, cookies, and sugar-laden cereals are just a few of the foods containing refined sugars. A glance at a label on a can of peas or other vegetable will often reveal that sucrose has been added. Salad dressings may contain refined sugar as an ingredient. For years even baby food contained amounts of refined sugars in foods that, if they contain any sugar at all, should have only naturally occurring sweeteners. Aware of the human preference for sweet-tasting foods, manufacturers intentionally include sweeteners in their products whenever they can—to appeal not only to the child, but to the adult who might taste the product as well. And it works. For example, while you may not be able to put your finger on why you prefer one bottled spaghetti sauce over another, if you read the labels, you will probably see that your preferred brand is the one with sugar added. As Martha Pehl, R.N., a representative of the Sugar Association, stated in an interview in 1979 when asked about the addition of sugar to products, sugar is "the catalyst that makes food eating pleasurable."[2] And intrinsically appealing.

As you attempt to diet, those foods that contain sweet products will appeal to you, and time and time again you will be impelled to choose them over the bland, the salty, the sour, or the bitter foods—

even though those foods may be just as filling and more nourishing. In order to resist the urge to yield to your instincts, you must first be aware of their existence and know when they are likely to assert themselves. Rarely is the first taste of a piece of pie or a cookie your last taste. The moment a sweet morsel hits your palate, your instinctive knowledge that it is a safe food encourages you to continue to eat.

THE INSTINCTIVE DRIVE FOR MEAT

It seems that modern man—a former hunter and gatherer—has been doing a little too much hunting at the meat counter and not enough gathering at the vegetable stand—all to his detriment.

Recent evidence shows that the modern diet has proved to be a bit too modern for the human body. Today's typical diet regimen (particularly in Western cultures such as ours) consists of an enormous amount of meat consumption as compared to the time when man was in the process of evolving. It is estimated that for a million and a half years, a meal by the entrance of the cave consisted of three times more plant food than animal food, particularly in tropical and temperate climates.[3] At the turn of this century protein in the form of animal meat only comprised a small percentage (thirty percent) of all protein eaten daily, and most people's diets consisted of much more carbohydrate (fruits, vegetables, etc.) and plant protein (nuts, beans, etc.). Today, however, there has been a dramatic increase in the consumption of animal protein. Food in the form of animal flesh accounts for seventy percent of the protein habitually consumed by Americans.[4] No meal seems to be quite complete or satisfying unless plates are piled high with the flesh (meat) of other animals: chicken, pork, beef, lamb, and fish. Yet, investigations into the eating habits of prehistoric man indicate that a meat-laden diet should not be the norm at all, and that now, in the 1980s, the consumption of large quantities of meat may be overloading the body's biological capacities.

Why has there been such an escalation in meat eating? Again, instinct is the culprit. After all, wouldn't you rather stalk and fell a deer in an hour, drag it back in one large, convenient "package" to your table, and live off its inherently high protein content for days, than spend an entire day wandering through the woods and fields, foraging for fruits, nuts, and berries, and expending tremendous amounts of energy for half a basket of low protein food?

Precisely! And in fact, it is suggested by archeologists, anthropologists, primatologists, and comparative anatomists, that although humans and their forebears were essentially herbivores (plant eaters), when meat was available, man eagerly helped himself, thus evolving into an omnivore.[5] Through happenstance, primitive beings found that not only was meat faster to obtain (particularly as hunting skills improved), but meat seemed to keep hunger at bay for many more hours than did vegetables. Also, primitive man realized he had a great deal more sustained energy after eating meat-covered chops or ribs than he did when he ate handfuls of berries. Naturally, early man did not know anything about caloric content of foods or about the relative merits of protein, carbohydrates, and fats, but he was quick to sense the benefits of one food over another when it came to satisfying his needs and enhancing his chances for survival. Also, anthropologists suggest that females, limited in mobility because of children and in strength because of build, but needing the nourishment that meat provided, began to align themselves with the "best providers" in the clan. The males, in exchange for sexual favors, began to provide extra meat for their women, and were encouraged to keep hunting by the women—or spend the night alone! Eventually, scientists theorize, vegetation became ranked lower as a food preference.

Of course, before man learned to herd his animals to create a ready food supply (an idea that developed over the course of many thousands of years), getting a choice piece of meat was mostly a matter of luck and opportunity. However, as part of his evolution, man has incorporated in his genes a kind of "thrift" mechanism that instructs him to take advantage of the situation when meat presents itself. Thus he developed his seemingly rapacious appetite for the flesh of other animals. This instinct—a survival mechanism—has carried over through generation after generation.

The following is a list of trends in the modern American diet. As you can readily see, animal flesh consumption has increased dramatically, as has consumption of food items containing sugar. Fresh vegetables have lost ground considerably.

FOOD TRENDS IN THE AMERICAN DIET

FOOD	TIME PERIOD	% CHANGE
Animal Flesh		
beef	1910–1976	+72
chicken	1910–1976	+388
fish (fresh and frozen)	1910–1976	+42
Vegetation		
fruit, fresh	1910–1976	−33
vegetables, fresh	1945–1976	−16
Sugared foods		
ice cream products	1910–1976	+1426
soft drinks	1960–1976	+157
sugar and sweeteners	1875–1976	+221

Source: Based on statistics from United States Department of Agriculture (Washington, D.C.: Center for Science in the Public Interest), 1978.

The Protective Instinct in Winter

Throughout the universe millions of cyclical patterns exist: the planets orbit the sun in a number of days that make up a specific planetary year, approximately 365 days for earth, and result in the seasons. Within this yearly revolution, the earth itself rotates on its axis, producing the patterns of light and dark that we know as days. Moreover, the inhabitants of our planet have their own internal cycles as a response to the various external cycles around them. When the sun goes down, nocturnal animals stir. As the dawn breaks they retire, and diurnal animals begin their activities. As the weather changes, reflecting the tilt of the earth on its axis and the position of specific latitudes relative to the warmth of the sun, creatures on earth begin the various adaptive processes that have enabled them to survive. Animals that must face a cold, bitter winter begin to produce longer protective hair, and in some animals their "winter coats" change color temporarily to blend with the snow-covered environment, thus enhancing chances for avoiding predators. In other animals, like most species of bear, the adaptive process causes them to hibernate.

Every species populating the planet today has developed its own adaptive processes, geared to help it through the good times as well as the bad. Some of the adaptive processes are unique to the particular species. Other adaptive mechanisms are universal, such as *an anticipatory weight gain just prior to winter months* combined with a metabolic mechanism that makes it very difficult to lose weight until winter is past.

Humans, like other animals, are imbued with genetic imprinting or instinct that causes biochemical changes to begin before winter descends. During the course of many thousands of years that have passed since man first migrated to colder regions of the globe, he has been able to survive *only* because each passing season an adaptive process was initiated that left him better prepared for the onslaught of winter.

Of course, eventually man brought his ever-increasing intelligence to bear on the problems of survival, and ultimately he learned to herd animals, grow plants from seeds, and store goods for the winter. Nonetheless, the years that passed prior to these innovations left him with an innate capacity to produce biochemical changes in his body that encourage him to eat and gain weight in anticipation for the winter season, and once that weight is gained, to slow down his metabolic rate to prevent rapid burning of excess body fat. Instinctively, your body senses that if it allows its stores of body fat to be depleted before the spring thaw ushers in new plant growth and the return of animals to the area, you might starve to death. Body fat requires far fewer calories to maintain itself than does muscle tissue. Once your body fat reaches a level of exhaustion that necessitates burning actual muscle for energy, your whole system enters a precarious state called starvation.

During the winter months, instinct is the culprit that makes it so difficult to shed extra weight. Even if you plan to fly to a tropical island and want to diet to fit into your bathing suit, bear in mind that, while you can succeed in taking weight off, your task may be more difficult than it would be in a different season. Although there are variations in the amount of winter weight gain people experience, just as there are subtle, instinctive differences between people whose ancestors were more concerned with seasonal drought or yearly monsoons than winter blizzards, each person comes equipped with instincts common to our species and refined by ancestral experience. We have no choice. It is in our genes.

NOTES

1. J. Descor, O. Maller, and R. Turner, "Taste Acceptance of Sugars by Human Infants," *Journal of Comparative and Physiological Psychology*, 84:1973, pp. 496–501.

2. "Contemporary Health Issues," Channel 10, Public Broadcasting System, Portland, OR, 10:30–11:00 AM, 13 February 1983.

3. Jane Brody, "Studies Suggest a Harmful Shift in Today's Menu," *The New York Times*, Science Times, 15 May 1979, Section C, p. 1.

4. Jane Brody, "Debate Cooking as US Acts on Nutrition," *Chicago Tribune*, 1 May 1980.

5. Boyce Rensberger, "Research Yields Surprises About Early Human Diets. Teeth Show Fruit Was Staple," *The New York Times*, Science Times, 15 May 1979, Section C, p. 1.

3

Body Design Dictates Diet

FACT: Your intestines have evolved to allow you to eat both vegetation and meat, but your teeth have remained geared best to vegetation.

FACT: You should greatly diversify your foods to fulfill dietary needs, lose weight, reduce cravings, and improve general health.

FACT: You are asking your body to digest chemicals that are completely alien to your system.

Take Your Cue from the Past

Evidence from the dim periods before recorded history began is incomplete, but as archaeologists sift through the thousands of centuries of rock debris, dusts, and deposits, the mystery of mankind continues to be unraveled. One of the most revealing findings is that, although man owes his special place among the world's species substantially to his relatively big brain and his complex nervous system, physiologically he has remained much the same as his more primitive ancestors. Though he may stand a little straighter and walk a little taller, today's human being has the same internal structure, layout, and design as his forebears millions of years ago. What has changed, however, is his food base, which is narrowing; the ratio of meat to plant material, which is increasing; and the unusual content of the foods he is eating, which more and more frequently includes substances that are not found naturally on earth, and that are completely foreign to his system.

14

LIGHTEN UP ON THE MEAT

Although preliminary studies by Dr. Alan Walker, an anthropologist at Johns Hopkins University, are based on only a few specimens of humanlike creatures, he has found evidence through electron microscope scanning of the teeth of *Australopithecus,* a forebearer of *Homo erectus* and *Homo sapiens* (you), indicating (through wear patterns) that fruit—alone—may have comprised earliest man's daily diet, and that the first indication that man had evolved into a plant and meat eater is with *Homo erectus,* the immediate ancestor of *Homo sapiens.*[1] This is also revealed by the structure of your teeth and your intestinal tract, which are different from those of other animals that rely totally on predation and meat for sustenance. True carnivores have large, sharp teeth to hold and kill their prey. You lack the large incisors that even your pet dog and cat have. Evolving as predators who needed the equipment to destroy and disembowel their victims, family pets, though now domesticated, still have the machinery to do the job. Some orthodontologists think tooth reduction and civilization are inseparable. Humans, as millions of years passed, developed the type of teeth that were less useful to bring down prey than they were to pry open shells, suck an occasional egg, and chew fruit from the trees and berries from the bushes.

Even the shape of your "human" face indicates that vegetation rather than meat was the norm. Most predators have long muzzles lined with sharp, pointed teeth (the better to eat you with), capped by highly sensitive noses (the better to catch your scent), whereas you have a truncated snout, large, flat back teeth and rather small, dainty eyeteeth. Muscle moves and shapes bone, and the fact that man's facial structure has evolved into what it is today indicates that he was essentially a vegetarian, grinding away at his food, rather than tearing at it. Eventually, the shape of man's jawline evolved through pressure from facial muscles to reflect the demands placed on the muscles used to chew. Cooked foods, easier to chew and therefore less work for jaw muscles, may also, it is hypothesized, have further changed man's facial structure.[2]

Your digestive tract also gives insight into evolved capabilities. Studies that compare and contrast the design of the digestive tract of the carnivore (meat eater), the herbivore (vegetable eater), and the omnivore (meat and vegetable eater) reveal that man was able to accept novel food, such as meat, and developed a kind of "combination" intestinal structure that allows for the digestion of both flesh and vegetation. Since meat putrefies much more quickly than vegetation, and the toxins produced can sicken the predator, carnivores have digestive tracts designed for quick processing of incoming food and rapid expulsion of waste material (as well as strong digestive enzymes better able to dissolve cartilage and bone).[3] Thus, the meat eater's digestive tract is short, smooth, and straight. The food gets eaten, digested, and expelled with dispatch before the animal becomes poisoned by his victim's decomposing flesh. Herbivores, on the other hand, have a small intestine and a large intestine that are lengthy and ideal for providing enough time for bulky, hard-to-digest foods to be broken down. Omnivores (which now include mankind) who eat grasses, vegetables, fruits, nuts, berries, as well as meat, have a digestive tract that is longer than the carnivore's, but shorter than the herbivore's. Puckered, rather than smooth, the surface area of the intestinal tract provides for a journey that is just long enough to digest the rougher items such as fruits, nuts, and berries, and just short enough to expel the animal flesh quickly before toxins become a problem.

INCREASE FOOD VARIETY

Humans are capable of eating much the same kinds and diversity of foods as other animals. In these modern times, we tend to forget that not so long ago man lived a much more basic existence, relying almost entirely on the immediate countryside and the variety it offered naturally, rather than trekking to the local grocery story or supermarket. Just like other creatures on earth, you eat leaves (spinach), stalks (broccoli), roots (potatoes, carrots, and onions), flowers (cauliflower), fruit (apples, oranges, bananas), seeds on grasses (rice, corn, wheat), seeds in pods (lima beans, peanuts, split peas) and beef, pork, chicken, fish, and eggs, or in some cannibalistic societies, each other. The difference is that man usually puts his food on a plate, whereas wild animals can be seen foraging and grazing in pursuit of the same fare.

In truth, like wild creatures, you could wander about a local woods and come across innumerable foods you could eat, if you had to, such as squirrels, rabbits, and porcupines, slugs and ants, dandelions, scarlet pimpernel, milkweed, and meadow garlic. An enormous amount of vegetation is edible to man. However, with the ease and convenience of supermarket shopping, much knowledge of available wild foodstuffs is now limited to folklore, those few survivors from another era who made the effort to document the vast variety available, and tribes such as the Seri Indians of the Sonora Desert in northwestern Mexico, who eat forty-one different kinds of fruit. In the *Journals of Lewis and Clark* (1804–1806) wild vegetable foods, common fare for the Indians, were totally foreign but of crucial importance to the survival of the American pioneers. As Thoreau wrote, "It takes a savage or wild taste to appreciate a wild fruit."[4]

OBTAINING A BALANCED DIET

Worldwide, it is estimated that there are thirty to fifty thousand edible plants available to embellish man's diet if he should want to avail himself of this variety. Yet most formulated foods contain more or less the same few ingredients. They may look different in texture, color, and flavor, but they are basically the same food. Coconut oil, for example, is the main ingredient in margarine, imitation nuts, chocolate, cheese, and nondairy creamers. The breakfast cereals lining shelf after shelf in the supermarket may have a multiplicity of flavors, but close inspection reveals that all consist of the same few grains. According to the April, 1982 *Consumer Reports,* products with a soy protein base account for 300 items sold in the average supermarket. Moreover, because agricultural practices artificially limit the diversity of vegetation that animals eat in their natural environment, food fed to livestock lacks variety as well.

Through a process of *food rotation,* wherein you do not eat the same food more frequently than once every four days, nor a food from the same family of foods more often than every other day (patterned after a diet devised by Herbert Rinkle, M.D., a highly respected pioneer in medicine), The 21st Century Diet is specifically designed to increase the variety and quality of foods you eat. That's not to say that you are going to be sent out into the wilderness with books about "back to nature" tucked under your arm and instructions not to return until you have filled a basket with fruits, nuts, and berries. Or that you'll be creating sandwiches out of the bark of the manzanita tree (edible though it is); rather, you will be noting and taking advantage of foods that are commonly available, though not necessarily found every day on your shopping list. The advantages of expansion of your food base will be threefold: first, you will discover what scientists have long known, that food variety protects health, and that consuming an increased amount of vegetation actually makes you feel better by eliminating the unnatural overload of meat products with which most of us have been burdening our systems; second, as a vital by-product of eating diverse foods, you will find that you increase the amount of vitamins and minerals taken into your body; and third, as discussed later, you will help yourself eliminate compulsive eating.

The following is a general list of foods available in the United States, broken into categories. A great deal of research has gone into the creation of this list, known formally as The Biological Classification of Foods. Based on original work by Warren T. Vaughan, a prominent American allergist, and modified by Alsop H. Corwin, Professor Emeritus of Chemistry at The Johns Hopkins University, The Biological Classification of Foods is the ideal guide to help you expand and diversify your diet. To those whose knowledge of botany and zoology is rusty, it may come as a surprise to discover that the tomato and the potato are considered to be in the same specific "family" of foods, as are the chicken and the pheasant. Classifications are no longer based on what grows underground or above ground. Biochemistry is now the deciding factor. Also, because plants and animals are now being examined and categorized based on biochemical criteria, rather than outward appearances, some fish have changed food families. For example, some "perches" are now "basses" and vice versa.

Glance briefly at the various food families and fill in the appropriate boxes with an "x." After you attain your weight goal, you'll be able to create your own menus and ensure you eat a balanced, vitamin-rich diet.

THE BIOLOGICAL CLASSIFICATION OF FOODS

	OFTEN EAT	RARELY EAT	CAN TRY	WON'T EAT
ANIMAL KINGDOM				
Amphibians				
Frog Family				
frog	——	——	——	——
Birds				
Dove Family				
dove	——	——	——	——
pigeon (squab)	——	——	——	——
Duck Family				
duck	——	——	——	——
eggs	——	——	——	——
goose	——	——	——	——
eggs	——	——	——	——
Grouse Family				
prairie chicken	——	——	——	——
ruffed grouse (partridge)	——	——	——	——
Guinea Fowl Family				
guinea fowl	——	——	——	——
eggs	——	——	——	——
Pheasant Family				
chicken	——	——	——	——
eggs	——	——	——	——
peafowl	——	——	——	——
pheasant	——	——	——	——
quail	——	——	——	——
Turkey Family				
turkey	——	——	——	——
eggs	——	——	——	——
Crustaceans				
Crab Family				
crab	——	——	——	——
Lobster Family				
crayfish	——	——	——	——
lobster	——	——	——	——
Shrimp Family				
prawn	——	——	——	——

THE BIOLOGICAL CLASSIFICATION OF FOODS

	OFTEN EAT	RARELY EAT	CAN TRY	WON'T EAT
shrimp	——	——	——	——
Fish (freshwater)				
Catfish Family				
catfish	——	——	——	——
yellow bullhead	——	——	——	——
Eel Family				
eel	——	——	——	——
Minnow Family				
carp	——	——	——	——
chub	——	——	——	——
Muskellunge Family				
Northern pike	——	——	——	——
pickerel	——	——	——	——
Paddlefish Family				
North American paddlefish	——	——	——	——
Perch Family				
sauger	——	——	——	——
walleye	——	——	——	——
perch, yellow	——	——	——	——
pike	——	——	——	——
Salmon Family				
salmon species:				
Atlantic	——	——	——	——
coho	——	——	——	——
dog	——	——	——	——
king	——	——	——	——
pink	——	——	——	——
sockeye	——	——	——	——
trout species:				
brook	——	——	——	——
brown	——	——	——	——
lake	——	——	——	——
rainbow	——	——	——	——
Smelt Family				
smelt	——	——	——	——
Sturgeon Family				
belugua	——	——	——	——

THE BIOLOGICAL CLASSIFICATION OF FOODS

	OFTEN EAT	RARELY EAT	CAN TRY	WON'T EAT
sturgeon caviar (granular)	——	——	——	——
Sucker Family				
bigmouth buffalofish	——	——	——	——
black buffalofish	——	——	——	——
sucker	——	——	——	——
Sunfish Family				
black bass species:				
largemouth	——	——	——	——
smallmouth	——	——	——	——
spotted	——	——	——	——
bluegill	——	——	——	——
sunfish species:				
longear sunfish	——	——	——	——
pumpkinseed	——	——	——	——
crappie	——	——	——	——
Whitefish Family				
lake whitefish	——	——	——	——
Fish (Saltwater)				
Anchovy Family				
anchovy	——	——	——	——
Barracuda Family				
barracuda	——	——	——	——
Bluefish Family				
bluefish	——	——	——	——
Codfish Family				
cod (scrod)	——	——	——	——
cusk	——	——	——	——
haddock	——	——	——	——
pollack	——	——	——	——
tomcod	——	——	——	——
Conger Eel Family				
conger eel	——	——	——	——
Croaker Family				
croaker	——	——	——	——
drum, red	——	——	——	——
sea trout	——	——	——	——
silver perch	——	——	——	——

THE BIOLOGICAL CLASSIFICATION OF FOODS

	OFTEN EAT	RARELY EAT	CAN TRY	WON'T EAT
spot	___	___	___	___
weakfish	___	___	___	___
Flounder Family				
dab	___	___	___	___
flounder	___	___	___	___
plaice	___	___	___	___
Grunt Family				
common	___	___	___	___
gray	___	___	___	___
yellow	___	___	___	___
Gurnard Family				
sea robin	___	___	___	___
sea tag	___	___	___	___
Halibut Family				
halibut	___	___	___	___
Harvest Family				
butterfish	___	___	___	___
harvestfish	___	___	___	___
Herring Family				
Atlantic	___	___	___	___
Pacific	___	___	___	___
sardine	___	___	___	___
shad	___	___	___	___
Jack Family				
amberjack	___	___	___	___
jack mackerel	___	___	___	___
pompano	___	___	___	___
yellow jack	___	___	___	___
Mackerel Family				
albacore	___	___	___	___
bonito	___	___	___	___
mackerel	___	___	___	___
skipjack	___	___	___	___
tuna	___	___	___	___
Marlin Family				
marlin	___	___	___	___

THE BIOLOGICAL CLASSIFICATION OF FOODS

	OFTEN EAT	RARELY EAT	CAN TRY	WON'T EAT
sailfish	___	___	___	___
Porgy Family				
scup (porgy)	___	___	___	___
Puffer Family				
puffer	___	___	___	___
Red Snapper Family				
red snapper	___	___	___	___
Sea Bass Family				
bass, yellow	___	___	___	___
grouper	___	___	___	___
perch, white	___	___	___	___
sea bass	___	___	___	___
Sea Catfish Family				
ocean catfish	___	___	___	___
Scorpionfish Family				
rosefish (ocean perch)	___	___	___	___
Shark Family				
shark	___	___	___	___
Silverside Family				
mullet	___	___	___	___
silverside	___	___	___	___
whitebait	___	___	___	___
Sole Family				
sole	___	___	___	___
turbot	___	___	___	___
Swordfish Family				
swordfish	___	___	___	___
Tarpon Family				
tarpon	___	___	___	___
Tilefish Family				
tilefish	___	___	___	___
Mammals				
Bear Family				
bear	___	___	___	___
Beaver Family				
beaver	___	___	___	___

THE BIOLOGICAL CLASSIFICATION OF FOODS

	OFTEN EAT	RARELY EAT	CAN TRY	WON'T EAT
Bovine Family				
beef cattle				
beef flesh and organs	_____	_____	_____	_____
milk products				
butter	_____	_____	_____	_____
cheese	_____	_____	_____	_____
dried milk	_____	_____	_____	_____
ice cream	_____	_____	_____	_____
yogurt	_____	_____	_____	_____
veal (young beef)	_____	_____	_____	_____
buffalo	_____	_____	_____	_____
goat (kid)	_____	_____	_____	_____
cheese	_____	_____	_____	_____
ice cream	_____	_____	_____	_____
milk	_____	_____	_____	_____
sheep (domestic)				
lamb	_____	_____	_____	_____
mutton	_____	_____	_____	_____
Rocky Mtn sheep	_____	_____	_____	_____
Deer Family				
caribou	_____	_____	_____	_____
elk	_____	_____	_____	_____
moose	_____	_____	_____	_____
reindeer	_____	_____	_____	_____
venison	_____	_____	_____	_____
Hare Family				
rabbit	_____	_____	_____	_____
Horse Family				
horse	_____	_____	_____	_____
Opossum Family				
opossum	_____	_____	_____	_____
Pronghorn Family				
antelope	_____	_____	_____	_____
Squirrel Family				
prairie dog	_____	_____	_____	_____
squirrel	_____	_____	_____	_____
woodchuck	_____	_____	_____	_____

THE BIOLOGICAL CLASSIFICATION OF FOODS

	OFTEN EAT	RARELY EAT	CAN TRY	WON'T EAT
Swine Family				
hog (pork)	___	___	___	___
bacon	___	___	___	___
ham	___	___	___	___
lard	___	___	___	___
pork gelatin	___	___	___	___
sausage	___	___	___	___
scrapple	___	___	___	___
Whale Family				
whale	___	___	___	___
Mollusks				
Abalone Family				
abalone	___	___	___	___
Clam Family				
clam	___	___	___	___
mussel	___	___	___	___
Octopus Family				
octopus	___	___	___	___
Oyster Family				
oyster	___	___	___	___
Scallop Family				
bay scallop	___	___	___	___
sea scallop	___	___	___	___
Snail Family				
snail	___	___	___	___
Squid Family				
squid	___	___	___	___
Reptiles				
Snapping Turtle Family				
snapping turtle	___	___	___	___
Diamondback Terrapin Family				
diamondback terrapin turtle	___	___	___	___
green turtle	___	___	___	___
Rattler Family				
diamondback rattlesnake	___	___	___	___

THE BIOLOGICAL CLASSIFICATION OF FOODS

	OFTEN EAT	RARELY EAT	CAN TRY	WON'T EAT
PLANT KINGDOM				
Banana Family				
banana	___	___	___	___
plantain	___	___	___	___
Beech Family				
chestnut	___	___	___	___
Birch Family				
filbert (hazelnut)	___	___	___	___
Buckwheat Family				
buckwheat	___	___	___	___
Carpetweed Family				
New Zealand spinach	___	___	___	___
Carrot Family				
carrot	___	___	___	___
celery	___	___	___	___
parsley	___	___	___	___
parsnip	___	___	___	___
Cashew Family				
cashew	___	___	___	___
mango	___	___	___	___
pistachio	___	___	___	___
Cactus Family				
prickly pear	___	___	___	___
Composite Family				
artichoke	___	___	___	___
chicory	___	___	___	___
endive	___	___	___	___
escarole	___	___	___	___
head lettuce	___	___	___	___
Jerusalem artichoke	___	___	___	___
leaf lettuce	___	___	___	___
Fungi Family				
mushroom	___	___	___	___
Goosefoot Family				
beet	___	___	___	___
spinach	___	___	___	___
Gourd Family				
cucumber	___	___	___	___

THE BIOLOGICAL CLASSIFICATION OF FOODS

	OFTEN EAT	RARELY EAT	CAN TRY	WON'T EAT
muskmelon	——	——	——	——
cantaloupe	——	——	——	——
casaba	——	——	——	——
crenshaw	——	——	——	——
honeydew	——	——	——	——
Persian	——	——	——	——
pumpkin	——	——	——	——
squash				
acorn	——	——	——	——
buttercup	——	——	——	——
caserta	——	——	——	——
cocozelle	——	——	——	——
crookneck and straightneck	——	——	——	——
cushaw	——	——	——	——
golden nugget	——	——	——	——
hubbard	——	——	——	——
pattypan	——	——	——	——
turban	——	——	——	——
vegetable spaghetti	——	——	——	——
zucchini	——	——	——	——
watermelon	——	——	——	——
Grass Family				
barley	——	——	——	——
corn	——	——	——	——
millet	——	——	——	——
oats	——	——	——	——
rice	——	——	——	——
rye	——	——	——	——
sugar cane	——	——	——	——
wheat	——	——	——	——
wild rice	——	——	——	——
Grape Family				
grape or raisin	——	——	——	——
Heath Family				
blueberry	——	——	——	——
cranberry	——	——	——	——

THE BIOLOGICAL CLASSIFICATION OF FOODS

	OFTEN EAT	RARELY EAT	CAN TRY	WON'T EAT
Honeysuckle Family				
elderberry	____	____	____	____
Laurel Family				
avocado	____	____	____	____
Legumes				
alfalfa (sprouts)	____	____	____	____
black-eyed peas	____	____	____	____
lentil	____	____	____	____
lima	____	____	____	____
mung	____	____	____	____
navy	____	____	____	____
pea	____	____	____	____
peanut	____	____	____	____
soybean	____	____	____	____
string	____	____	____	____
Lily Family				
asparagus	____	____	____	____
chives	____	____	____	____
garlic	____	____	____	____
leek	____	____	____	____
onion	____	____	____	____
shallot	____	____	____	____
Mallow Family				
okra (gumbo)	____	____	____	____
Miscellaneous				
honey	____	____	____	____
Morning Glory Family				
sweet potato	____	____	____	____
Mulberry Family				
fig	____	____	____	____
mulberry	____	____	____	____
Mustard Family				
broccoli	____	____	____	____
Brussels sprouts	____	____	____	____
cabbage	____	____	____	____
cauliflower	____	____	____	____
celery cabbage	____	____	____	____

THE BIOLOGICAL CLASSIFICATION OF FOODS

	OFTEN EAT	RARELY EAT	CAN TRY	WON'T EAT
Chinese cabbage	____	____	____	____
collard greens	____	____	____	____
kale	____	____	____	____
kohlrabi	____	____	____	____
radish	____	____	____	____
rutabaga	____	____	____	____
turnip	____	____	____	____
watercress	____	____	____	____
Myrtle Family				
guava	____	____	____	____
Olive Family				
green olive	____	____	____	____
Palm Family				
coconut	____	____	____	____
date	____	____	____	____
Papaya Family				
papaya	____	____	____	____
Pedalium Family				
sesame seeds	____	____	____	____
Pineapple Family				
pineapple	____	____	____	____
Pomegranate Family				
pomegranate	____	____	____	____
Potato Family				
eggplant	____	____	____	____
green pepper	____	____	____	____
pepino	____	____	____	____
potato	____	____	____	____
tomato	____	____	____	____
Protea Family				
macadamia nut	____	____	____	____
Rose Family				
Pomes				
apple	____	____	____	____
crabapple	____	____	____	____
pear	____	____	____	____

THE BIOLOGICAL CLASSIFICATION OF FOODS

	OFTEN EAT	RARELY EAT	CAN TRY	WON'T EAT
Stone Fruits				
almond	——	——	——	——
apricot	——	——	——	——
cherry	——	——	——	——
nectarine	——	——	——	——
peach	——	——	——	——
plum (prune)	——	——	——	——
Berries				
blackberry	——	——	——	——
dewberry	——	——	——	——
loganberry	——	——	——	——
raspberry	——	——	——	——
strawberry	——	——	——	——
Rue (Citrus) Family				
grapefruit	——	——	——	——
kumquat	——	——	——	——
orange	——	——	——	——
pomelo	——	——	——	——
tangelo	——	——	——	——
tangerine	——	——	——	——
Sapacaya Family				
Brazil nut	——	——	——	——
Saxifrage Family				
gooseberry	——	——	——	——
Sedge Family				
Chinese water chestnuts	——	——	——	——
Spurge Family				
tapioca	——	——	——	——
Walnut Family				
black walnut	——	——	——	——
butternut	——	——	——	——
English walnut	——	——	——	——
hickory nut	——	——	——	——
pecan	——	——	——	——
Yam Family				
Chinese potato (yam)	——	——	——	——
yampi	——	——	——	——

ACQUIRING A TASTE FOR NEW FOODS

A study of the food preferences of 128 preschoolers, their parents, and unrelated adults indicated that though food preference could not be radically changed, it could be modified by parents. Liking or disliking a food is partly a matter of what is culturally acceptable and typically eaten by people of the same ethnicity. Food preference is based on cultural influences passed down from generation to generation. In China, for example, there was a widespread aversion to cow's milk. Although cow's milk made "scientific sense," it offended the "cultural sense" of the Chinese, and they rejected it.[5] In Africa, Australia, South America, New Guinea, and Japan, grasshoppers (and locusts) are eaten . . . and ounce for ounce contain twenty percent more protein than dried beef!

Halvah, chutney, and tripe are delicacies to some people, yet practically inedible foods to others. In those instances when you think you or members of your family will not appreciate or even entertain the thought of eating new foods you select, bear in mind that your own parents introduced you to less familiar foods such as spinach, prunes, and liver a little at a time until you "acquired" a taste for these items. Yes, you turned your nose up at first, but later accepted—even came to prefer—some of these foods. When you introduce new and seemingly "exotic" foods in your menus, use the same method.

People invariably prefer the foods with which they are familiar. After a little exposure, attitudes can change and in time eschewed foods may be considered quite palatable. Often a little periodic tasting is the answer (a good reason to encourage variety when children are young).

Though these foods may be unusual to you, The 21st Century Diet encourages you to expand your food horizons . . . and try them. Cookbooks abound that will help the neophyte in unchartered supermarkets. No need to buy a "plantain" only to discover it is not an unripe banana! Get out of the habit of pushing the shopping cart only down certain aisles or the habit of cooking only certain meals.

As you saw in The Biological Classification of Foods, there are many foods from which to choose. Although not all plants and animals may be indigenous or available in your area, your grocery shelves certainly offer a much wider variety of foods and food families than you probably are in the habit of eating. Diversify! Cut down on red meat! The recommended daily allowance is approximately 44 grams per day for a woman and 56 grams per day for a man, or *one* generous-sized hamburger a day. Yet the typical American eats an average of 106 grams per day, and of that 71 grams is animal protein. You'll find that your meals not only become more interesting but more nutritious as well, because variety promotes health. As you approach The 21st Century Diet plan that is appropriate for you, keep these suggestions in mind. When you complete the first phase of The 21st Century Diet and turn to the last chapter to create your own menus, you will discover a richness in eating that will surprise you. Yes, it will take a little creativity, and even some effort as you "shop around," but it will be worth it . . . and pay dividends in helping you to maintain your new svelte figure and your newfound agility.

NOTES

1. Boyce Rensberger, "Research Yields Surprises About Early Human Diets: Teeth Show Fruit Was the Staple," *The New York Times,* Science Times, 15 May 1979, Section C, p. 1.

2. Lloyd B. Jensen, *Man's Foods* (Illinois: The Garrard Press, 1953).

3. Kim Hill, "Hunting and Human Evolution," *Journal of Human Evolution,* vol. 11, no. 6 (September 1982), pp. 521–544.

4. Oliver Perry Medsger, *Edible Wild Plants* (New York: MacMillan, 1966).

5. "Editor's Comments," *Journal of Nutrition Education,* vol. 13, no. 1, Supplement 1981.

4

Keeping "Diet" Time with Your "Inner Clocks"

FACT: Your morning coffee makes you *more* tired than when you first woke up, evening coffee keeps you awake, and coffee between the hours of 3:00 and 4:30 in the afternoon has *absolutely no effect* at all.

FACT: You can lose more weight faster if you consume most of your daily calories *before* four o'clock in the afternoon.

FACT: Your breakfasts and lunches must contain protein or you will be tired and hungry throughout the day.

FACT: Your supper should consist of predominantly high carbohydrate foods if you are to lose maximum weight and sleep well in the process.

Dieting to the Beat of Your Own Daily "Rhythms"

Every day about dawn your body begins a biochemical cycle that signals the "active" period of your day. You stir under your covers in anticipation of waking. If you have set an alarm clock, often you reach over and silence its potential noise a split second before it goes off. Whether you live on a farm, in the suburbs, or in the city, whether you rely on an alarm clock or on your "inner clock" to wake you, as a creature who has evolved into a daytime animal over the millennia, you have no choice; you must follow a preordained program that is part of your genetic programming.

Some of the program commands are second by second, minute by minute, hour by hour. Others are day by day, week by week, month by month, year by year. The goal of the program or rhythm is to keep all your systems functioning separately and yet in synchrony. Although your mind is the master clock, within each cell in your body there is a individual "clock" that affects the cell's timing. Ultimately, all the rhythmic patterns (and there are billions of them) work together not only to make sure you breathe, blink your eyes, swallow, urinate more during the day than at night, enter adolescence, and become capable of reproduction; but also to provide mental acuity and physical prowess during the daytime and to lower body temperature and lessen alertness and metabolism at night so you can sleep. These body rhythms (not to be confused with so-called "biorhythms," which have absolutely no scientific basis) play a crucial role in The 21st Century Diet.

Getting to Know Your Body Rhythms

Dr. Charles F. Ehret, senior scientist at The Argonne National Laboratory just outside Chicago, Illinois, has described the cycles of body rhythms as being so dramatic that throughout a single day "it is as if you were a blond at night and a redhead at dawn."[1] So different can you be, biochemically, throughout the course of twenty-four or twenty-five hours (a circadian day*) that in some instances your reaction to drugs and medications can "cure" you if taken at the "appropriate" time or potentially "kill" you if taken at the "wrong" time. (For years, in fact, researchers at the University of Minnesota have known that chemotherapy for cancer victims varies in effectiveness depending upon what time of day the patient is exposed to the therapy.)[2]

In much the same way, though with less severe consequences, your biochemistry reacts to the food you eat each day. These reactions change depending upon what you eat and when you eat it. Digestion and metabolic rate have cyclical patterns, too. Not only are hunger pangs cyclical, letting your body know when it is necessary to eat, but digestive enzymes are also released at regular intervals to make it possible for you to absorb nutrients from the foods you eat. In addition, your metabolic rate changes, burning off

*The term *circadian* is derived from the Latin words "about" (*circa*) and "day" (*dies*). Franz Halberg, M.D., during his research at the University of Minnesota, noticed rhythmic fluctuations in white blood cells of laboratory animals over the course of a day. It was Halberg who defined these rhythms as circadian.

calories less or more efficiently depending upon what time of day it is, what month it is, and how old you are.

THE CASE FOR HIGHER PROTEIN BREAKFASTS AND LUNCHES

Man is built from and fueled by the food he digests. His skeleton, muscles, organs, blood, hair, fingernails, etc., are essentially just a reorganization of the recycled water, protein, fat, carbohydrate, and salts that he consumes and that are miraculously transformed into his own unique, human form.

After thirty years of research by scientists specializing in chrono-biology (the study of how time affects living organisms) it is now known that the digestive enzymes man releases during the morning and afternoon best utilize *protein*, whereas, the chemicals released in the evening best digest *carbohydrates*.[3] Over the ages your body evolved to process protein best during the daylight hours because you need a great deal of energy during the day when you are active, and a meal consisting predominantly of high protein foods (fish, eggs, dairy products, beans, meat) has the ability to guarantee you up to five hours of sustained energy by stimulating natural chemical changes in the adrenalin pathway in your brain cells. Carbohydrates, however, can only provide you with approximately one hour of increased energy, after which your energy level plummets to a point even lower than before eating anything at all. Carbohydrates (vegetables, fruit, pasta, desserts) tend to affect the indoleamine pathway in the brain, and put you to sleep.

Take a look at the following illustrations. The first one compares the effect of eating protein, carbohydrates, and fat on blood sugar (or your energy levels). Notice how carbohydrate and fat cause a sudden surge of blood sugar levels over the course of an hour, but immediately thereafter, actually cause fatigue. Protein, even though it takes about two hours to have an energizing effect that equals that of carbohydrates, ultimately provides your body with a steady source of energy upon which it can draw for hours. The second illustration highlights the different sources of protein that can be used to generate sustained energy. Note that plants as well as animals can provide you with the kind of long-lasting energy that a busy day requires.

EFFECT OF PROTEIN, FATS, AND CARBOHYDRATES ON BLOOD SUGAR LEVELS

You need energy during the day, and protein (meat, eggs, dairy products, fish, nuts) supplies what you need by causing an increase in your blood sugar—or energy—levels. The higher the level, the more energy you will have. In the evening carbohydrates (pasta, desserts, alcoholic beverages, vegetables) will ensure a good night's sleep. (*Adapted from Dr. Raymond Green,* Human Hormones *[London: Weidenfeld and Nicholson, 1970], p. 232.*)

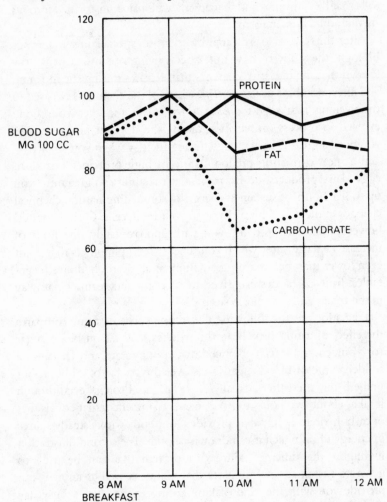

THE PROTEIN GROUPS

Energy-generating protein is found in a variety of plants as well as in animals. Legumes, grasses, seeds, and nuts provide the same type of long-lasting energy boost that milk products, eggs, and meats offer. Although the sources are different, the results are the same. When counting on having a busy, demanding day, be sure to plan on a source of energy on which you can count—protein.

GROUP I
PLANT PROTEINS

1. Legumes (beans and peas)
   black, kidney, red, pink, pinto, cottage, navy, mung, lima, black-eyed, garbanzo (chick peas), peanuts, lentils, soybeans
2. Grasses
   barley, bulgur, corn, oats, rice, rye, triticale, wheat
3. Seeds and Nuts
   pumpkin, sesame, walnuts, pecans, almonds, cashews, coconut, pinenuts, pistachio, sunflower

GROUP II
ANIMAL PROTEINS

1. Milk products
   milk, cheese, yogurt
2. Eggs
3. Meats
   poultry, fish, beef, lamb, pork

Based on this information, the typical breakfast fare of black coffee and a piece of toast with, perhaps, a half of a grapefruit, qualifies as just about the *worst* possible food combination with which to begin the day. Eat that type of breakfast and you are virtually guaranteed to feel fatigued . . . and to suffer the onslaught of the hunger pangs that accompany depleted energy reserves.

THE CASE FOR HIGHER CARBOHYDRATE SUPPERS

Since protein foods provide you with hours of energy, if you eat a big steak at supper time your natural tendency to fall asleep in the evening hours will be disturbed. However, if you sit back and enjoy a plate of pasta covered with tomato sauce (meatless), have a glass or two of red wine, and top it all off with a sweet dessert, you will have no trouble sleeping at all. According to Dr. Ehret, a world-renowned authority on man's circadian rhythms and on *dyschronism* (circadian rhythms gone awry as a result of rapid transcontinental travel or of work schedules that involve shifts "around the clock"), one remedy is to make sure you eat hearty, predominantly high protein breakfasts and lunches, and almost entirely high carbohydrate suppers. In this way your circadian rhythms fall back into their natural synchrony, providing a great deal of energy during the day and a waning of energy at night.

The 21st Century Diet is geared to take these circadian rhythms into account. Meals are formulated on a predominantly high protein breakfast and lunch plan, and a predominantly high carbohydrate supper plan. In this way while on your diet you are assured of sustained energy throughout the active hours of your day, and guaranteed a sound night's sleep once your day is done.

THE CASE FOR MONITORING CAFFEINATED BEVERAGES

You get up in the morning, stagger to the kitchen, turn on the coffee maker, and wait for the rich aroma to fill the house or apartment. It's ready! All across America and around the world men and women start their days with a cup of hot coffee (or tea). It's practically a way of life. Yet, what most people do not realize is that *methylated xanthines,* an "umbrella term" covering chemicals that include caffeine and theobromine, found commonly in coffee, and theophylline, found naturally in many teas, have the ability to affect you differently at different times throughout the day. Consumed in the morning, methylated xanthines set your body clock *back*. Consumed at night, methylated xanthines set your body clock *ahead*. Thus, in the morning, the cup of coffee you drink to stimulate you can actually decrease your energy. Shortly after you finish the cup of coffee, the chemicals begin to affect your body clock. The same "inner clock" that woke you up the hour before, now gets a clear message from the methylated xanthines to let you go back to sleep.[4] If you add cream or sugar to your coffee, the carbohydrates and refined sugar conspire to give you a brief increase in energy, and then they join the methylated xanthines to sap your energy. Similarly, at night the coffee again affects your biochemistry profoundly. Only this time it tricks your body clock into thinking it is dawn, with the end result that you have trouble sleeping because your "active" cycle has been triggered. *Only* between the hours of 3:00 and 4:30 in the afternoon do methylated xanthines leave your body clock unaffected.

Dr. Ehret discovered this phenomenon while studying methods to help shift workers (firemen, nurses, doctors, assembly line workers) adapt to varying schedules that might include working through the night. Since working when you would normally be asleep requires an adjustment of the body clock, Dr. Ehret searched for ways to help make this adjustment more rapid. He discovered that methylated xanthines were very powerful chemicals that had a dramatic effect on the "timing" of body clocks. By charting the effect of methylated xanthines on body clocks throughout the course of a day, he was able to determine just when the appropriate time was for a shift worker to use coffee to help him or her make the body clock time change. The by-product of this research is new insight into problems associated with drinking coffee or tea with caffeine in the morning, throughout the day, and in the evening.

Why doesn't coffee affect you in the afternoon? Dr. Ehret is not sure. He only knows that it has to do with your biochemistry and being more or less susceptible at different times of the day and night. (Alcoholic beverages also have different effects on the human biochemistry throughout the course of a day. A martini at dawn is much more likely to be felt than at dusk.)

If you want to drink coffee, do, but pay attention to the clock. In the morning coffee is *not* a stimulant. At night, if you want to sleep well, drinking coffee after dinner is a big mistake. On the other hand, if you have to stay up late for whatever reason, drink coffee! Eat a higher protein supper! You should have all the energy you need.

The following is a list of items containing the methylated xanthines in the form of caffeine. Note that they are not limited to coffee. Tea, diet soda, candy, and drugs can also contain methylated xanthines. Indeed, many more items contain methylated xanthines than you might suspect.

METHYLATED XANTHINES (CAFFEINE, THEOBROMINE, THEOPHYLLINE) CONTENT OF BEVERAGES AND DRUGS

PRODUCT	QUANTITY	METHYLATED XANTHINES (MILLIGRAMS)
Coffee		
decaffeinated	5 oz.	2
instant, regular	5 oz.	53
percolated	5 oz.	110
drip	5 oz.	146
Tea		
one-minute brew	5 oz.	9–33
three-minute brew	5 oz.	20–46
five-minute brew	5 oz.	20–50
canned iced tea	12 oz.	22–36
Cocoa and Chocolate		
milk chocolate	1 oz.	6
cocoa beverage	6 oz.	10
baking chocolate	1 oz.	35
Nonprescription Drugs		
stimulants		
Caffedrine capsules	standard dose	200
NoDoz tablets	standard dose	200
Vivarin	standard dose	200
pain relievers		
plain aspirin	standard dose	0
Anacin	standard dose	64
Midol	standard dose	65
Excedrin	standard dose	130
diuretics		
Pre-Mens Forte	standard dose	100
Aqua-Ban	standard dose	200
Permathene	standard dose	200
cold remedies		
Coryban-D	standard dose	30
Triaminicin	standard dose	30
Dristan	standard dose	32
weight-control aids		
Dietac	daily dose	200
Dexatrim	daily dose	200
Prolamine	daily dose	280

Source: Consumer Reports, October 1981.

CAFFEINE CONTENT OF *SUGAR-FREE* SOFT DRINKS
(Milligrams per 12-ounce can,
as determined by *Consumer Reports* tests)

Diet Mr. Pibb	52	Diet Pepsi	34
Tab	44	Diet 7-Up	0
Diet Dr. Pepper	37	Diet Sunkist Orange	0
Diet Rite Cola	34		

Source: Partially adapted from *Consumer Reports,* October 1981, p. 599.

The 21st Century Diet encourages you to regulate your intake of all foods, beverages, and drugs that contain methylated xanthines. The diet plans allow for decaffeinated coffee and herbal tea anytime, and caffeinated coffee and plain tea only between the hours of 3:00 and 4:30 in the afternoon. If you think you simply cannot function without a cup of coffee in the morning, and that you are "addicted," try giving coffee or tea up just for a day or two. By rescheduling your caffeine intake you will allow your body clock to reestablish its normal cycle, instead of being slowed down repeatedly in the morning and speeded up in the evening. Thus, although The 21st Century Diet is primarily designed to help you control body weight, adopting The 21st Century Diet regimen also permits you to improve your overall health by stabilizing your body rhythms. So *don't* turn the coffee pot on in the morning . . . and *do* eat predominantly high protein breakfasts and lunches, and predominantly high carbohydrate dinners, and you will be well on your way to rapid weight loss . . . and renewed health.

THE CASE FOR EATING HIGHER CALORIE FOODS BEFORE 4:00 P.M.

In 1974, in an experiment at the University of Minnesota Medical School, seven people (four men and three women) were placed on a one meal per day regimen for two weeks. During the first week the one meal per day was eaten as a breakfast meal at 7:00 A.M. Throughout the second week the one meal per day was switched to 5:30 in the evening. Each meal consisted of exactly 2000 calories. The results of the experiment revealed that *timing* of food intake was a major factor in weight control. During the first week when the men and women were eating their meal in the morning, *everyone* lost weight—approximately 1 1/4 pounds each. During the second week, however, when meals were consumed in the late afternoon, all but one person realized a weight *gain* of almost a pound. If this amount does not sound too impressive, bear in mind that there are 52 weeks in a year. If the men and women had continued to eat 2000 calories a day in the early evening, extrapolation would indicate a 52 pound weight gain in one year! Looking at it another way, assuming your weight is currently stable, if you were to consume the majority of your calories before evening, you could potentially lose up to 9 pounds in one month without any radical change in the types of foods you are eating. (This study, by the way, was presented at the 12th Conference of the International Society for Chronobiology in Washington, D.C., in 1975. Its authors included Franz Halberg, M.D., and thirteen of his colleagues.)

In today's hustle-bustle society, rarely (except perhaps on Sunday) do people sit down to a hearty breakfast anymore. Yet, based on your body's energy demands throughout the morning and into the afternoon, breakfast should supply at least one-fourth to one-third of your daily calorie requirements. If you are like most people, chances are your breakfast is very light and contains more carbohydrate than protein. Lunch, an equally important meal, is skipped by as many as one in five people every day.[5] More often than not it's a case of sleeping as late as possible, rushing to get dressed, taking a quick sip of orange juice and possibly a piece of toast—or not stepping into the kitchen at all. As your grandmother and possibly even your mother probably told you, breakfast is important. In fact, it is vital for several reasons: to replenish energy levels, to stave off distracting hunger pangs, and to permit optimal mental and physical function.

Over the course of the night your energy level has dropped and needs replenishing. For all intents and purposes your "tank" is on "empty." A predominantly high protein, high calorie breakfast actually enhances your ability to concentrate and perform by giving you a steady and sustained boost to your energy level for the next several hours. If you go out without breakfast, or even worse, eat foods that are predominantly high in carbohydrates (fruit) or that are laden with sucrose (refined sugar in cereals, jellies, a sweetened cup of coffee) you actually deplete your energy supplies even further. In addition you are left with prelunch hunger and fatigue. Hunger is reflected in the body by physical contractions of the stomach. Over fifty years ago the scientist Tomi Waada discovered that these contractions take place about every one and a half hours and are an instinctive signal to keep "foraging," even though people in today's society have graduated to more sophisticated methods of putting food on the table. If you skip breakfast, in particular, you will find these instinctive reminders less a suggestion than a direct order.

Quite simply, your body needs food to function optimally. Since more demands are placed on energy levels during the course of your active day, it is wise to anticipate those needs and fill them by giving your body what it wants—high protein food in the morning and afternoon.

BREAKFAST LIKE A KING. LUNCH LIKE A PRINCE. SUPPER LIKE A PAUPER.

The 21st Century Diet is designed to take your circadian rhythms into account by providing you with a diet plan that has you consuming most (51 percent or more) of your calories before supper and by making the meals predominantly high in protein. That does not mean you will be barely eating an evening meal, however. On the contrary, there will be a great deal of food offered that you may eat at supper time. However, most of it will be high carbohydrate and low calorie. You won't miss eating "in quantity." The total volume of food you eat each day will depend upon the specific plan you choose to follow. Follow that program and you will be filled with energy during the daytime, will sleep well at night . . . and will lose a great deal of weight in the process.

NOTES

1. Charles F. Ehret, Ph.D., and Lynne Waller Scanlon, *Overcoming Jet Lag* (New York: Berkley Publishing Group, 1983), p. 54.
2. Ibid., p. 31.

3. Gay Gaer Luce, "Biological Rhythms in Psychiatry and Medicine," U.S. Department of Health, Education, and Welfare, Public Health Services, DHEW Publication No. (ADM)78–247, 1970, p. 52.

4. Charles F. Ehret, Ph.D., K. R. Groh, and J. C. Meinert, "Considerations of Diet in Alleviating Jet Lag," *Chronobiology: Principles and Applications to Shifts in Schedules*, L. E. Scheving and F. Halberg, eds. NATO Advanced Study Institutes Series (Maryland: Sijthoff and Noordhoff, 1980), p. 394.

5. William Gatty, *The Body Clock Diet* (New York: Simon and Schuster, 1978), p. 124.

5

It's Often a Family Affair

FACT: You are probably not the only overweight person in your family.

FACT: You are overweight primarily because of the type and quantity of food that your parents put on the table rather than an hereditary predisposition toward gaining weight.

FACT: You do not have a genetic flaw that results in your gaining weight, but *where* you will put weight on is hereditary.

FACT: Your desirable weight has more to do with muscle-to-fat ratios than standard height/weight tables.

How Much Should You Weigh?

Who knows best how much you, as an adult, should weigh? Opinions vary significantly on this subject. What to one person appears excessive, to another may appear voluptuous. Weight, within reason, often is less a medical classification than a cultural judgment. In addition, there is a great deal of conflicting information on the relative advantage or disadvantage of being slightly underweight or slightly overweight. Dr. Reubin Andres, clinical director of the National Institute on Aging, reviewed forty studies concerning the possible relationships between weight and longevity. Dr. Andres determined that men and women weighing from fifteen to twenty percent more than the weight recommended by insurance company tables tended to outlive men and women in the same age group who were considered the "right" weight by the charts. Yet, the federal government Health and Nutrition Examination (HANES) suggests that your ideal weight should be determined by how much you weighed in your twenties. HANES recommends that you maintain that weight, whatever it was, throughout your adult life. All very confusing, particularly if you are not now in your twenties or you were terribly under- or overweight during that decade.

The Metropolitan Life Insurance Company recently released an updated version of their very popular height/weight chart. Based on a twenty-two year "mortality rate" study of the longevity of over four million healthy adults, it was discovered, as Dr. Reubin Andres determined, that heftier people appeared to have a better chance at a longer life than thinner people. In response to this data, Metropolitan Life updated the old figures on their 1959 height/weight charts to reflect a more generous weight allowance, particularly for shorter people. A small-boned 5'2" woman, according to the new height/weight charts should weigh between 128 and 134 pounds. A large-boned man standing 5'6" may tip the scales at between 140 and 159 pounds. To many people these allowances are far too high, and will be rejected immediately because, as Dr. Paul S. Entmacher, medical director of Metropolitan Life says, the new charts do not take into account a person's sense of his own ideal weight in terms of appearance.[1] Nor do the charts reveal the types of advanced medical measures that may have gone into saving the lives of men and women (whose statistics comprised the study) who might otherwise have died from accidents or diseases—regardless of their weight. Richard Simmons, a formerly obese actor who turned successfully to diet and exercise to keep weight down and stay in shape, and who has an enormously successful health-oriented TV show, responded to inquiries by the press about the new height/weight charts by saying, "I'd throw myself in the river," if he found himself weighing in at 151 pounds (the maximum allowed for a medium-framed man of 5'6"), instead of his usual 134 pounds.[2] The sentiments, no doubt, of the millions of his weight-conscious viewers.

The Metropolitan Life height/weight charts for men and women do have a few problems—not the least of which is that the designers of the chart seem to think that men and women weigh themselves while fully dressed and wearing shoes with "one-inch heels." (Perhaps this is a throwback to the days when bathroom scales were not the norm and people had to weigh themselves on public scales for a penny!) However, the real problem with these and many other height/weight charts is that they do not base their recommendations on "ratio of muscle to fat." Arnold Schwarzenegger, the body builder, has massive muscles that add many pounds to his weight, but because he is lean (meaning he has very little extra fat on him) he is not considered overweight at all. Ruthi Shafer, a 5'2" twenty-three-year old who has won outstanding weight-lifter awards for two years in a row in national finals, can dead-lift 479½ pounds. Pure muscle, she weighs in at 132 pounds.[3] Yet persons the same height as Schwarzenegger and Shafer may weigh the same, but instead of being lean, would be flabby and fat. In addition, the height/weight charts assume that everyone has either a small, medium, or large frame, when a simple glance at a room full of people will reveal that bodies are more often a mix. A person can be barrel-chested and yet have bird-like legs. You could have a tiny waistline and be small and fine boned from the waist up, but big-hipped and heavy-legged from the waist down.

MUSCLE-TO-FAT RATIOS

Ideally, in your early twenties you should have approximately 18 percent body fat if you are female and 12 percent body fat if you are male; ratio of fat to muscle differs with gender because the female of the species has natural hormones that encourage the storage of body fat against future needs of pregnancy. (Very overweight men and women often have up to 50 to 60 percent body fat!) Since the aging process automatically tends to increase body fat, as you get older you have to work a little harder at maintaining muscle tone so that what you've got continues to look good, and does not become supplanted with fat. For example, at age 20 you could have weighed 120 pounds and had the ideal amount of body fat. At age 30, however, even if you did not gain a pound, your percentage of body fat would have increased of its own accord, possibly to 25 percent or more. By the time you are 40 years old, it is entirely possible that, while still weighing the same, your body could consist of 35 percent body fat. A slightly discouraging but not insurmountable situation!

Bear in mind, also, that muscle weighs more than fat. Therefore, you can be at the "maximum" desirable weight *only* if you are in good physical shape. If you are not very active and have a "soft" body, meaning your weight disproportionately favors fat, rather than muscle, then you should opt to weigh the "minimum" recommended amount. That way you will be thin and look trim, even though you won't be considered "toned."

There are several ways to assess your muscle-to-fat ratio. One of them involves the use of a calibrator that resembles the pincers on a lobster. The calibrator grabs and measures folds of flesh at strategic places around your body. There is also a "hydrostatic" approach that requires you to expel your breath and be submerged in a tub of water. Through mathematical calculations, professionals are able to determine your percentage of fat. An easier method is to measure the girth of your calf to get a rough estimate of your muscularity. (Height does not count.) The following is a good guide for dieters who are only one to twenty-five pounds overweight, but bear in mind that you should have a fairly proportionate frame to use this method; if you are top-heavy or bottom-heavy, the results won't be as accurate.

CALF GIRTH MEASUREMENT

DEGREE OF ESTIMATED MUSCULARITY	WOMEN	MEN
Poor	12½" and less	14" and less
Average	12½" to 13½"	14" to 15½"
Excellent	13½" and more	15½" and more

Of course, the age-old at-home method that still works is to strip down and stand on the bathroom scale. If you cannot bear the thought of seeing your actual weight registered, an alternative that some people prefer is simply to watch their naked silhouette change in the mirror as the days go by. Diet until you like the silhouette you see. (But don't go too far. The anorexic look should not be the goal!) Ideally, you should aim to diet away all your extra fat and exercise your way to toned muscles. As a general guideline, refer to the table below. If you are flabby and have a poor degree of muscularity, you should weigh less than if you are toned and have a high degree of muscularity. Ultimately, you must determine your best weight on the basis not only of calibrations, but also on how you look and feel and whether you are participating actively in an exercise program that is replacing fat with muscle. Note that the ideal weight tables for men and women represent flat-footed height and birthday suit weight.

IDEAL WEIGHTS FOR MEN
Based on 12% Body Fat and Degree of Muscularity

HEIGHT	POOR MUSCULARITY	AVERAGE MUSCULARITY	EXCELLENT MUSCULARITY
5'2"	135	141	149
5'4"	141	147	155
5'6"	147	153	161
5'8"	153	159	167
5'10"	159	165	173
6'0"	164	171	179
6'2"	170	177	185
6'4"	176	183	191
6'6"	182	189	197
6'8"	188	193	203

IDEAL WEIGHTS FOR WOMEN
Based on 18% Body Fat and Degree of Muscularity

HEIGHT	POOR MUSCULARITY	AVERAGE MUSCULARITY	EXCELLENT MUSCULARITY
5'0"	94	100	106
5'2"	102	108	114
5'4"	110	116	122
5'6"	118	124	130
5'8"	126	132	138
5'10"	134	140	146
6'0"	142	148	154
6'2"	150	156	162
6'4"	158	164	170

Fat Runs More in Households Than in Genes

The predisposition toward where on your body you store excess weight may be hereditary, but the fact that you are overweight appears to be more a result of the particular eating habits of the people who raised you. In a study reported in *Ecology of Food and Nutrition,* investigators discovered that 147 children who were *adopted* often resembled their adoptive parents in relative weight.[4] Overweight parents, more often than not, create overweight children, as the parents' eating habits become part of the child's. (Interestingly, the same holds true for pets. *The Veterinary Record,* in 1970, published an article called "Obesity in Pet Dogs" by E. Mason. The article revealed that overweight people overfed their dogs, too.)

Of course, all people have traits and characteristics that are passed along via the genes through heredity. Height, eye and hair coloring, bone structure, tone of skin, etc., are all part of your bill of lading when your parents produce you. The biochemical ability to utilize food more efficiently may also be an hereditary factor, but, again, it seems more often to be a case of what your parents have put on the table to eat.

Who's Responsible for the "Shape" You're In?

THE HEREDITARY FACTOR IN BODY SHAPE AND FAT DISTRIBUTION

The inherited "mix" of disparate bone structures is a fairly recent phenomenon in evolutionary time spans, and is the result of a blend of body types. Originally, frames evolved as a method to enhance survival. In different parts of the world (which were very isolated geographically until man developed a means of rapid, long-distance transportation) environmental conditions tended to increase the chance of survival of those animals who could best adapt. In a world where food, water, oxygen, and warmth spelled the difference between life and death for prehistoric man, natural selection ("survival of the fittest") tended to weed out those animals that failed to adjust to their environment. The relationship of physique to climate follows certain ecological rules. People from tropical climates tend to be slighter and lighter in weight than those living in areas of the country where temperatures can become frigid. A small person can sweat more efficiently and his water and salt requirements are less than those of a larger, heavier person. It is even suspected that facial features reflect the environmental conditions from which the person's ancestors evolved. Noses, for example, tend to be more open-nostriled in humid places where there is much moisture in the air. Yet, in the desert and extremely cold parts of the world, where air is extremely dry and moisture is at a premium, native peoples tend to have a more closed, narrow nose opening. Based on this phenomenon, anthropologists theorize that the nose evolves in a particular shape to help hold drier air more efficiently in order to extract the most moisture from it.[5]

Invasion, war, migration and immigration, as well as ease of transportation, have resulted in offspring that reflect different phenotypes (species with collective characteristics). Whereas at one time entire populations of one area of the world tended to be similar in build, color, and body type, now the distinctions are less clear, and result in a variety of physical types and constructions. These separate parts come together to form a "compromise" human being in much the same way cross breeding of livestock (Black Angus cows and Jersey cows, or greyhounds and German shepherds) produces characteristics that are a blend. It is not so easy to spot a child with stereotypical physical traits of a Northern European (tall, blond) if he or she has a parent or grandparent or great grandparent who was Mediterranean by descent. Similarly, it can often require more than a glance to determine if someone is of Irish descent, though there are still people with the stereotypical red hair. Human mating among a variety of cultures has produced offspring with a mix of physical conformations: large shoulders, short legs, or fine bone structure combined with enormous height, for example.

Bone structure or conformation is hereditary, and there is nothing you can do about being fine-, medium-, or heavy-boned—or about your particular pattern of fat distribution or "genetic predisposition" to gain weight in your face, thighs, waistline, etc. If you have a large derrière and heavy legs, look around, somebody else in your natural family does, too. You do not have to be obviously overweight to discern that your natural parents' "lines" have passed down to you, either directly from one parent or as a mix of inherited bone structure and musculature from both.

Generally, as illustrated on the following page, fatty deposits for the human species tend to occur in certain specific areas of the body, but genetic programming plays a crucial role in determining where the most weight gain will occur. Some people have a tendency to gain more weight from the waist down, or the waist up, or develop huge bulging stomachs. "Cellulite," a nonmedical term popularized commercially by Nicole Ronsard, a French dietician, is simply a massing of fatty deposits. Although there is a controversy about the methods required to eliminate cellulite, the general consensus is that a diet that burns off fat (and fatty deposits are fat) and changes the ratio of muscle to fat in favor of muscle will dramatically reduce the puckered skin under which the fatty deposits lie. Also, some authorities feel that exercise makes fatty deposits more mobile, distributing them more evenly throughout the body.[6]

Your Overweight Child

T. J. Coates and his colleagues reported in *Addictive Behavior* in 1978 that overweight children ususally have overweight parents. The children of obese parents were significantly fatter "at all ages" than the children of average weight or lean parents.

Bearing in mind that parents control the food intake of their preschool children and the majority of the meals of their elementary, junior high school, and high school offspring, the study suggests that parents must assume responsibility for controlling the weight of

PRINCIPAL FAT DEPOSITS

Fatty deposits tend to gather in specific areas of the body. Distribution, however, can be greatly influenced by genetic programming. If one of your parents has a tendency to concentrate weight gain in the hips, or waist, or under the chin, there is a good chance you inherited the same predisposition toward a preponderance of extra fatty deposits in that same area.

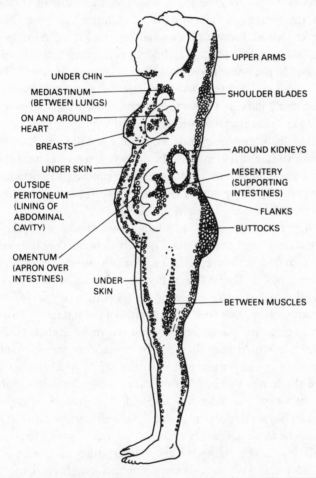

UPPER ARMS

UNDER CHIN

MEDIASTINUM
(BETWEEN LUNGS)

SHOULDER BLADES

ON AND AROUND
HEART

BREASTS

UNDER SKIN

AROUND KIDNEYS

OUTSIDE
PERITONEUM
(LINING OF
ABDOMINAL
CAVITY)

MESENTERY
(SUPPORTING
INTESTINES)

FLANKS

BUTTOCKS

OMENTUM
(APRON OVER
INTESTINES)

UNDER
SKIN

BETWEEN MUSCLES

Source: Fad Diets Can Be Deadly by Frank Netter, M.D. © Frank Netter, M.D. Reprinted by permission of the author.

their children. In a recent study, again reported by T. J. Coates and his colleagues (this time in *The American Journal of Public Health*), third and fourth graders were given lectures in good nutrition, followed by an analysis of the children's lunches. As the lecture series progressed and the children became more and more aware of what constituted a sound nutritional approach to diet, the content of their lunch boxes began to change. Rewards in the form of stickers, buttons, rubber stamps—all emblazoned with the logo of the Stanford Heart Disease Prevention Program—provided sufficient "positive reinforcement" to sustain the children's enthusiasm for adjusting their diets. On the home front, the children began to influence their parents' decisions about what to prepare for the lunch boxes. A follow-up study indicated that the impact of the educational process persisted long after the study was completed.

As an adult, by changing your approach to quality meals and by using positive reinforcement (also possibly referred to as mild bribery for a good cause) to encourage your children to participate willingly, you have an excellent chance of modifying their behavior and reducing their overall weight problem.

The only real concern lies in finding out what it will take to motivate your youngster to follow The 21st Century Diet approach. The key is to find out what it is he or she really wants. For example, at a meeting of The Young Presidents Organization in New York, a psychologist told the story of how he tried to motivate his two young sons to keep their rooms clean without constantly importuning, threatening, and punishing. As a last resort, he announced that if the children would keep their rooms immaculate for six months without any carping on the part of either the phychologist or his wife, the children would be given brand new bicycles in the spring, six months away. The older boy responded by instantly springing into action. No shoe was out of place. No wrinkles appeared in his bed, which he made religiously every day. His closets were in perfect order. His books were stacked neatly on their shelves. The other boy, however, continued his slovenly ways, rarely making his bed, tossing his clothes on the floor at will, and wallowing in the general disorder of his room. At the end of the six month period a family conference was called in which the older boy was, as promised, given his new bicycle. Dismayed that he could not in good conscience give his younger boy a new bicycle also, the father threw up his hands and lamented his disappointment in his younger son. "But Dad," the boy said, "if you had only offered me a puppy . . . "

You have to know what it will take. Offer the wrong reward and you won't get the desired results. Ask your child. For some children it will be the promise of a material item, a doll, train, a bicycle. For others, it will be cold hard cash—money for the toy store, the movies, a tank of gasoline.

The other approach you can take to get your child started on a weight loss program is to enroll him or her in a camp. It need not be a "fat farm." Almost any camp will do. Regulated eating, and limited portions combined with increased physical activities, will create an atmosphere guaranteed to shed pounds. The camp does not have to be one specializing in overweight children—unless your child is extremely overweight. In that instance, children not being known for their tactfulness to one another, it might be better to consider the program designed specifically to eliminate the psychological problems often inherent in a situation where one child is greatly limited in his athletic ability due to excessive weight. Camp is supposed to be fun, not an ordeal.

When the child returns from camp, he will have established a new routine, and can be much more easily led into The 21st Century Diet. Since athletic prowess should have been enhanced at camp, continue the exercise aspect by signing your child up for activities at the "Y" or intramural games after school. Keep the momentum up . . . and the pounds will come down.

Which plan (800, 1200 or 1600 calories) should your child be placed on? Growing children need many more calories each day than a person who has attained his adult height. First, determine your child's ideal weight. (Ask your pediatrician if you are unsure.) Second, note the illustration below, which outlines energy requirements per pound of body weight in calories for children. If your child should weigh about 100 pounds and is 12 years old, multiply 16 (the energy requirement per pound of body weight in calories) × 100, and put him or her on The 21st Century 1600-calorie plan.

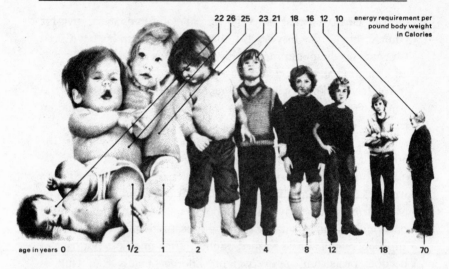

If your child is still growing, you must determine his or her daily basic caloric needs on a different basis from that of a person who has reached adult height.

Source: From *Atlas of the Body and Mind.* Copyright © 1976 by Mitchell Beazley, Ltd. Published in the U.S. by Rand McNally and Company.

Getting Everybody on The 21st Century Diet Program

Very often, criticism comes from the one person who thinks he or she has less of a problem than the others. Yet, studies have revealed that if food addiction, instinctive slowing down of metabolism, or lifestyle change does not affect you, simple aging will. Therefore, dieting is a family affair.

The best approach is to tackle the problem as a family, either passively or actively. (If you live alone, you can create your own support system with roommates, classmates, friends, or even contact a family member and try The 21st Century Diet together, even if it is only to compare notes over the telephone.) It is patently unfair to receive criticism for being overweight, be expected to do something about it, and have family members refuse to participate in what is essentially a family problem, particularly if they are less than perfect specimens of physical fitness themselves.

If you look around your dining room table and see family members who are also overweight, have a family discussion that emphasizes not only the weight reduction aspects of The 21st Century Diet, but the need for group participation among family members. And remember, dieters with spousal cooperation prove to persevere more easily while on a diet and manage to keep the weight off longer, too.[7] In your discussion highlight the following:

1. Determine the cause of the weight gain you or other members of your family has experienced. Every member of your family will experience some weight gain from the age factor. Those who have experienced new jobs, new careers, new babies, or other changes may also be struck by added weight. Those family members who have been on again off again dieters will recognize themselves, and since addictive food allergy runs in families also, that may be the root of the problem. You could easily have a combination of problems. Nonetheless, The 21st Century Diet will help family members lose weight, and not gain weight in the future.

2. Resolve to change eating patterns to conform to the 21st Century Diet: predominantly high protein breakfast and lunches, and predominantly high carbohydrate suppers. Explain that the shifting of emphasis from heavy, high carlorie, high protein meals at night will help prevent weight gain in a family with a predisposition to be overweight and will be a tool for weight reduction among family members already too heavy.

3. Discuss the immediate advantage to the entire family of consuming the majority of calories earlier in the day, when most of the energy is needed anyhow, and during which time calories are more efficiently burned.

4. Discuss the rotation aspect of the program. Let the family in on the research behind the suggestion not to eat the same foods too frequently, as described in Chapter Seven. Explain that cravings disappear when the same food is not eaten too often, and that allergies of all kinds, including the addictive kind, lift markedly when the rotation method is employed.

5. Let it be known that, while the family is not going to be reduced to carrying peanuts around to serve as their main source of protein,

protein intake in the form of animal flesh will be reduced and other forms that fill the human body's requirements will be found. Consumption of red meat will drop (too many calories, too many grams of protein in one 3-ounce portion), poultry consumption will rise, and fish will more frequently be part of a meal. Nuts and various high protein beans will also make an appearance.

6. Reassure family members that because of the 800-, 1200-, and 1600-calorie plans, they will still have plenty to eat and will be satisfied after each meal.

7. Get a consensus among family members about activities in which they could participate as a group or individually in order to attack extra weight by burning additional calories as well as regulating their consumption—and what it will take to motivate each person. (Werner Wolf, the sportscaster, commented recently about a baseball player whose weight was constantly ballooning. His inability to control his weight became such a problem that he was offered $7000 by his team manager if at every home game he weighed in at 215 or less. There were eleven more home games scheduled that season. The Aga Khan may not be motivated to diet with that kind of incentive, but most people would find that $7,000 or $77,000 would provide the fortitude necessary to keep under 215 pounds. To each his own motivation!

8. Emphasize that you are talking about a group effort, not a one-man stand. If they do not think they have a problem, let them acknowledge that you do and ask them to begin to work as a caring family to help you and any other overweight members. In this way they, too, become responsible for the success of your diet.

Now that you have determined how much you should weigh, it is time to determine the *cause* of your excess weight. As is explained in the following two chapters, there are three categories into which most overweight people fall. The first category involves *creeping weight gain*, the second category includes people who experience *rebound weight gain*, and the third category encompasses men and women who suffer from a problem known as *food addiction*.

There is a questionnaire in the next chapter to help you pinpoint the reason for your weight gain. Since food addiction is a severe problem (often associated with enormous weight gain), if you fall into that category, there is an entire chapter devoted to how to break food addiction—forever. First, however, answer the questionnaire.

NOTES

1. "Keep Your Double Chins Up," *Newsweek,* 14 March 1983, p. 65.
2. Ibid.
3. Howie Stalwick, "Weights No Burden to 132-Pound Ruthi," *The Oregonian,* 10 March 1983, p. 12.
4. S. M. Garn, P. E. Cole, and S. M. Bailey, "Effect of Parental Fatness Levels on the Fatness of Biological and Adoptive Children," *Ecology of Food and Nutrition,* vol. 16 (1976), pp. 91–93.
5. Yehudi A. Cohen, *Man in Adaptation* (Chicago: Aldine Publishing Company, 1974).
6. Barbara Edelstein, M.D., as quoted in "The Waist-Away Bikini Diet—4 Weeks to a Wonderful Figure," *Harpers Bazaar,* May 1982, p. 123.
7. K. D. Brownell, et al, "The Effect of Couples Training and Partner Cooperativeness in the Behavioral Treatment of Obesity," *Behavior Research and Therapy,* 16:323–33, 1978.

6

The 1 to 25 Pound Problem

FACT: You can gain weight from *natural causes* due to aging.

FACT: You can put on weight from a change in your daily routine.

FACT: You can experience ballooning of weight because of too frequent or too severe dieting.

The Great Weight Gain Conspiracy

At some time or another almost everyone seems to fall victim to weight gain. Indeed, the odds are that even those people who were almost painfully thin as youngsters will wake up one morning, look in the mirror and, to their surprise, realize they, too, have a weight control problem. Sometimes the problem can be directly attributable to metabolic programming as part of the aging process. Other times the reason is a critical change in daily schedule that results in a significant decrease in activity level. Occasionally, the situation may even be the result of too much dieting too often. Since all three factors are not mutually exclusive, often the problem of weight gain is a combination punch.

The following questionnaire should help you pinpoint the origins of your weight gain problem. Ask yourself if you fall into one of these categories:

QUESTIONNAIRE:
IS YOUR WEIGHT GAIN FROM "NATURAL CAUSES"?

	YES	NO
1. Have you just passed another decade?		
2. Have you just attained your adult height?		
3. Have you recently become pregnant?		
4. Have you just had a baby?		
5. Have you just begun college?		
6. Have you just begun a full-time job?		
7. Have you recently become more affluent?		
8. Have you recently retired?		
9. Have you been injured?		
10. Have you a debilitating ailment?		
11. Have you become a recovering alcoholic?		
12. Have you been sporadically dieting?		
13. Have you experienced headache, fatigue, weakness, depression, irritability, etc., upon being late for or missing a meal?		
14. Have you noticed you go on eating binges or food jags?		
15. Have you kept food on your nightstand ready for a middle-of-the-night snack?		
16. Have you taken diet pills and found they do not seem to work?		

If you answered "yes" to one or more of these questions, then your weight problem is completely understandable . . . and also entirely predictable! If you responded "yes" to questions 13–16, you may have a serious problem known as "food addiction," which is explained in detail in the next chapter.

The following sections elaborate on the specific factors that allow or cause weight to sneak up on you, appear virtually overnight, or continually reappear despite your efforts to maintain your weight goal. To diet effectively you should know the types of situations that might arise in the future or that might well be part of the problem today.

Creeping Poundage

CALORIC NEED CHANGES OVER THE COURSE OF YOUR LIFETIME

Weight gain is invariably everybody's problem. It's just a matter of time. As you grow older, you can expect to gain weight—even if you have never varied the amount of food eaten by even one calorie. Increasing age = decreasing metabolic rate = increasing weight.

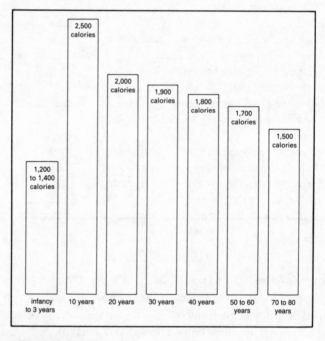

THE AGE FACTOR

If, throughout the course of your life, you never varied the number of calories that entered your body each day, you would still tend to gain weight. The aging process and its inherent biochemical changes take a toll in insidious weight gain. Slowly, often subtly, always relentlessly, as the decades slip by you can expect to gain weight. In fact, the director of the Obesity Research Clinic at St. Lukes Roosevelt Hospital in New York anticipates a weight gain of up to twenty-seven pounds as you grow older.

As you age, your brain begins to orchestrate hormonal changes within you as part of a natural process. Your muscle-to-fat ratio changes, in favor of fat. Body fat needs fewer calories than muscle to maintain itself. If you fail to anticipate these hormonal changes and devise a plan to compensate for them, you will gain weight; it is inevitable. Since your metabolism (in effect, your furnace) is being ordered hormonally to slow down—by as much as thirty percent from the time you are in your midtwenties until you are in your forties, fifties, and sixties—you gradually grow not only heavier but "softer," as toned muscle gives way to increased fat. This accounts for why, when you look in the mirror, you see sagginess, rather than firmness, and why you often have to work harder than ever to tone up (and replace fat with muscle). Even if you have not gained a single pound, your weight has changed in composition.

Sudden Weight Gain

CHANGE-IN-LIFE-CYCLE FACTORS

Occasionally, for no apparent reason, you experience a rapid gain in weight. It might surprise you because you may never have had a problem with excessive weight before or you thought you had conquered the problem for life. Following are some of the changes in circumstances that people experience periodically throughout their lives that result in rapid weight gain. If you have suddenly gained weight, chances are you will fit into one of the categories listed below.

1. You've recently completed your adolescent growth period. If you are a first-time dieter, then you now know the shock of realizing that you, too, have a problem. Your growth has tapered off and your hormones have begun to stabilize, yet you are still eating as fast and furiously—and in as much quantity—as you were when your body required extra calories to provide you with the energy and vitamins and minerals needed to help you attain your adult height. Perhaps you no longer participate in a school sport. Suddenly, those highly caloric sandwiches after school, washed down with a quart of whole milk, followed by endless snacks after supper, have stopped being burned, and are beginning to pile up. You have filled out and out . . . and out. In young women, in particular, the lean tomboy look gives way to a rounder, more cushioned (with fat) look in physical anticipation of possible pregnancy and the need for stored fat. Often it is quite startling to see the difference in weight from one year to the next in "aging" adolescents.

2. *You recently gave birth or are nursing.* The minute you become pregnant, your body undergoes tremendous changes as it provides a biochemical and physical accommodation for your fetus. Fat storage begins in anticipation of nine months of *in utero* nurturing. As your baby gains body weight, every time you step on the scale that additional weight is being recorded along with yours. Since women tend to rely heavily on the bathroom scale, the mirror, and the fit of clothing for indicators of unwanted weight, pregnancy totally disrupts personal weight monitoring techniques. Yes, your doctor checks your weight gain; however, with a distorted silhouette as well as an inability to see your toes (let alone read the bathroom scale digits as the months progress) each and every familiar restraint is gone for at least nine months. Up go the pounds—your baby's and yours.

Nursing mothers have to deal with carrying extra weight as well. Up to ten pounds of extra fluid is retained in order to be converted into mother's milk for the infant. Once again, mirror, scale, and clothing become useless aids to keeping slim.

3. *You recently began college.* Whether you are fresh out of high school or were graduated years ago and have decided to continue your education, you are about to experience a change in your daily schedule that will require you to spend a great deal of time sitting down. Unless you are also an athlete while in college and therefore involved in strenuous exercise, the requirements for scholastic achievement will necessitate not only sitting for many hours in class, but sitting behind your own desk at home to study. All that studying may do wonders for your brain, but it causes real problems with the shape of your derrière.

Also, if you have moved out of your family home and are living in an apartment or on campus, you may find your eating schedule has changed as well. If you are no longer restricted to eating three meals a day (perhaps prepared by someone else), the quality as well as the quantity of your daily food intake may alter. You may snack more often, eating on the run from one class to a next. Often those "quick" foods are filling . . . and fattening.

4. You have entered or reentered the job market. Whether it's your first job or a return to work after many years of being out of the job market, when you start, much like the new student, you will have to establish a new daily routine. Unless you are working at a job that requires a great deal of physical exertion, such as construction work, you will find yourself spending almost your whole day immobilized at a desk. Other than moving down halls and around office furniture, the only real exercise you may get during the week may be periodic trips to the snack cart. "Secretarial spread" can be endemic . . . and not limited to those sitting behind a typewriter.

5. You have become more affluent. If there is a sudden change in the economic climate in your house, whether that means the children have grown up and departed or are self-supporting, or your employer has given you a substantial raise, or you have reached the time of life when you can afford to take it a bit easier, you will find that you upscale accordingly, and this finds expression as weight gain. Perhaps you are no longer mowing your own lawn once a week, someone else is; some trim, slim youngster from the neighborhood, no doubt. Or if you used to walk the children to the park for recreation in order to supervise their play, they now may walk to the park without you or take your car to the local mall to have fun. More often than not you find you are less physically active than you used to be around the house. Perhaps you eat out more now, and indulge yourself in food and drink much more than you did when you had more financial restrictions. With increased affluence, unless you watch your food and drink intake carefully, you gain weight.

6. You have reached retirement age. Retirement may be a wonderful change in your life, but it is often accompanied by unwanted weight gain. Four decades of research show that when humans suddenly become inactive, they spontaneously fatten up. Although being able to "sleep in" at last may sound delightful, often not having a scheduled day results in doing almost nothing. Even if you were very active on the weekends during the years that you worked, expanding those activities to fill the weekdays may not always be possible. Moreover, if your typical weekend during your work years was to relax and do as little as possible, you are going to see a dramatic change in weight.

Those years after retirement can also be affected by age-related diseases and infirmities. These, too, can slow you down and complicate the weight maintenance problem. The answer, of course, as in any dramatic change in daily schedule, is to try to compensate. If you don't, you will see your waistline expand in direct proportion to your inactivity.

7. You have suffered an injury. Depending upon the severity of your injury, your recuperation time can become a period of unanticipated weight gain. If you are incapacitated for weeks or months or years on crutches, in braces, or in a wheelchair, you can expect a significant change in your mobility and your ability to burn calories efficiently enough to maintain your preaccident weight. You may be biding your time until your injury heals by eating excessively, more out of boredom than anything else; if so, a short amount of time monitoring your intake should be all that's necessary. If the extent of your injury is such that you will never be able to resume your former activities fully, you will have to initiate a radical change in your eating habits.

8. You have developed a chronic ailment. Any illness (or disease) that forces you to lead a more sedentary life, even if only temporarily, can lead to weight escalation. For example, arthritis can affect your ability to remain active, as can angina or diabetes. If you have an ailment that limits mobility, unless you fight against letting the problem overwhelm you, the cycle always becomes a vicious one: the worse you feel, the less you get out; the less you get out and work to maintain what strength you do have, the more debilitated you get; the less you exercise, whether you have increased your daily caloric intake or not, the more weight you gain.

9. You have given up smoking cigarettes. Many people can attest to the problem of soaring weight gain after having stopped smoking cigarettes. The feeling of malaise that begins from the moment you deny yourself a cigarette seems to be alleviated only by eating food.

In reality, the desire for food in place of a cigarette has nothing to do with hunger, per se; rather it is a misdirected attempt to stave off nicotine withdrawal symptoms and chemical withdrawal symptoms that feel vaguely like hunger pangs.

The problem is that cigarette withdrawal symptoms last an inordinately long time. Not only are you addicted to the nicotine, but to the chemicals in the cigarettes as well. Along with nicotine, there are literally hundreds of manmade chemicals in cigarettes: tobacco is sprayed with poisonous insecticides, the dried tobacco leaf is treated with chemicals to impart flavor, and lamps filled with kerosene are used to keep tobacco plants warm during cold spells. All of these chemicals leave a residue that gets incorporated into the tobacco leaf, the smoke from which in turn gets drawn into your lungs . . . and within a few seconds, into your bloodstream, chemicals and all.

During the months it can take to break the addiction to nicotine and eliminate the chemical residues from your body, withdrawal symptoms continue to masquerade as feelings of hunger, sending you to the refrigerator time and time again. In addition, authorities theorize that the chemicals in cigarettes affect your basal metabolism rate, speeding it up when you habitually smoke and slowing it down when you suddenly stop smoking. The result of a slowed metabolism, combined with constant eating is, of course, enormous weight gain.

10. You have recently married. You used to eat and run or eat large meals only when you dined out, but now you and your spouse spend the evening hours indulging in a large meal together every night. One mate takes great pride in preparing the supper and the other eats everything on his or her plate, if not simply because the food is delicious, but out of a sense of obligation or to avoid hurt feelings. The net result is that you both begin to gain weight and suddenly find yourselves in clothes that strain at the seams. As a note of interest, male spouses seem to set the weight tone for the household. Researchers R. W. Jeffry and R. R. Wing found that, if the husband allowed himself to gain weight, it was just a matter of time before the wife lost control of her weight, too. But if the husband was conscientious about keeping his weight under control, the wife was less likely to gain.[1]

Single adults generally live a less homebound life than couples.

The refrigerators and kitchen cabinets of single people often reflect the amount of importance that organized meal planning plays in their lives. Indeed, researchers have found that there is a distinct relationship between your relative body weight and the quality and quantity of food stored in the home. Virtually bare refrigerators and cabinets are often the norm during single years if people are trim, whereas, when you have a mate, you tend to stockpile his or her "favorite" foods, as well as those that will be needed to complete a balanced meal. The open, half-empty can of tuna that was the sole inhabitant of the refrigerator gives way to shelves bursting with foodstuffs.

Rebound Weight Gain

CHRONIC WEIGHT GAIN FACTOR

Frank Dobinsky, a New Englander, has lost more than 1000 pounds over the last twenty years. In his most recent effort, he lost 100 pounds, then "ballooned up past 300 pounds."[2] Constant dieting actually promotes weight gain. Richard Keesey, Ph.D., psychologist at the University of Wisconsin, placed laboratory rats on a starvation diet until the rats reached eighty-one percent of what would have been considered normal rodent weight. When taken off their starvation diet, the laboratory rats overcompensated for their drastic diet by gaining twice as much weight as they had lost during the imposed starvation. Survival instincts were to blame.

One of our natural instincts is to provide a method to help survive when food is in short supply. When you go on a drastic diet or eat one meal per day, your instincts do not know it is *you* who is limiting the number of calories or meals; your instincts respond as if some uncontrollable circumstance, such as a volcanic eruption or an earthquake, has made food and game scarce. Because your instinct is programmed to help you survive this disaster, it acts to slow your metabolic rate down and burn fat reserves very, very slowly. Your body, uncertain as to how long the famine will last, understands it must hang onto its fat reserves because fat takes fewer calories to maintain than lean muscle. That is why everything you eat "seems to turn to fat," and often, as Dr. G. Bray said in *The Obese Patient* (New

York: Saunders Co., 1976), people who eat the least number of meals each day appear to fight the most difficult weight battles. If instinct permitted fat to be burned up, your body would require one-third to one-half *more* calories a day to maintain muscle. So it grabs and stores whatever food it can get. Repeated dieting *trains* your body to prepare for long periods of scarcity.

Of course you are not consciously aware of this protective process going on within you, but it is operating, nonetheless. When food suddenly appears to be abundant and the "hard times" seem to be over, instinct makes you eat more than usual so that you actually surpass your previous weight and build up even more reserves than you had before the "famine." Compounding the problem is the fact that your metabolic rate, now in a lower "emergency" gear, continues to burn fat slowly until it seems safe to resume the usual rate. During that whole period, you are gaining weight.

Yes, rebound weight may be your problem. However, also bear in mind that inaccurate calorie counting may be a factor as well. At Queen Elizabeth College in London, twenty-nine women who claimed not to have been able to lose weight when on a 1000–1500 calories per day regimen were isolated and placed on a strictly monitored 1350 calories per day diet. Each day the women were weighed prior to breakfast. One week later only ten of the twenty-nine still had not lost weight. Nineteen, however, had obviously failed to keep accurate records before.[3]

What about the other ten? They confirmed the slowed metabolism theory. Psychologists Susan and O. Wayne Wooley, professors at the University of Cincinnati College of Medicine, had obese patients record every single morsel of food they ate each day. The Wooleys discovered that their overweight patients ate what would be considered normal or even less than normal amounts of food each day. Two patients, in particular, managed to maintain more than 260 pounds of weight on 1000 calories per day. Seems impossible? Yet it was obvious that the metabolic rates of these people were turned so far down that losing weight was impossible. Their metabolic rates were so slow, it was surmised, because overweight people are chronic sporadic dieters who suffer periodic severe food deprivation as they attempt to lose weight. Their bodies were trying frantically (and successfully) to avoid sudden semistarvation states by automatically turning down the rate of metabolism.

Compounding the problem is the fact that fat requires far fewer calories to maintain than muscle. You can need from one-third to one-half fewer calories to maintain your fat than a lean person needs to maintain muscle. In a study of 100 high school students reported in the March 1983 issue of the *Journal of the American Dietetic Association,* those young women who were overweight consumed an average of only 1,203 calories each day, barely enough caloric intake to maintain the weight of an 88-pound women at age 65, let alone a more active teenager.[4]

The good news is that in other tests comparing the metabolic rates of fat people as compared to lean people, once fat is lost through diet (or by diet and exercise), metabolic rate can stabilize.[5]

Whether you are the victim of creeping weight gain, sudden weight gain, or rebound weight gain, The 21st Century Diet will enable you to diet successfully. Although the various factors that caused your weight gain will also affect the course and duration of your diet, anyone and everyone can take off unwanted pounds. It is just a case of knowing what caused the weight gain and what to do about it. The 21st Century Diet has the explanations and the solutions.

NOTES

1. T. J. Coates, R. W. Jeffry, and R. R. Wing, "The Relationship Between Persons' Relative Body Weight and the Quality and Quantity of Food Stored in Their Homes," *Addictive Behavior,* 3:178-84, 1978.

2. Laura White, "The Promise of a Slimmer You Fades with Fad Diets," *USA Today,* 8 March 1983, p. 4D.

3. D. S. Miller and S. Parsonage, "Resistance to Slimming: Adaptation or Illusion?" *Lancet,* 5 April 1975, pp. 773-75.

4. "Heavier Girls Eat Less Food," *Sunday Oregonian,* 27 March 1983, p. LC27.

5. Michael A. Dunn, Sharyn K. Houtz, and E. W. Hartsok. "Effect of Fasting on Muscle Protein Turnover, the Composition of Weight Loss, and Energy Balance of Obese and Non-obese Zucker Rats," *The Journal of Nutrition,* vol. 112, no. 10 (October 1982), pp. 1862–1875.

7

The 25 + Pound Problem

FACT: You can gain weight from unnatural causes due to an addictive form of food allergy.

FACT: You can break food addiction with a four day program.

FACT: You *must* free yourself from food addiction before beginning The 21st Century Diet.

Compulsive Overeating

It is almost your bedtime and, as you contemplate turning in for the night, you meander toward the refrigerator where your nightly snack is waiting. In fact, every night, without fail, you look forward to the same snack. Nothing else will quite do. So you open the refrigerator door and, much to your dismay, you find either that you are out of your favorite snack or someone else has eaten it. What do you do? Do you simply turn in for the night—a little disappointed— or do you put your coat on and head for the nearest neighborhood all-night delicatessen?

If you would not hesitate to head out into the night, then you have what is commonly referred to by bioecologists as *food addiction*. Far different from the weight increases associated with aging, a change in your daily schedule, or constant dieting, the weight that is gained due to food addiction results from a biochemical dependency not unlike drug addiction.

Everyone knows about the type of food allergy that produces hives, rashes, nausea, or diarrhea, but few people, including quite a

71

few allergists, realize that there are actually three types of allergies: *cyclical allergies* that come and go, *fixed allergies* that always cause a problem, and *addictive allergies* that create a physiological dependency on the very food that is causing the allergy.[1] As in any addiction, when the substance to which you are addicted is removed, you experience withdrawal symptoms. With the addictive form of food allergy, withdrawal creates physical and mental symptoms that seem completely unrelated to allergy, and, therefore, are often completely misdiagnosed. The physical symptoms include chronic fatigue or general weakness, trembling or heart palpitations, regular or migraine headache—any problem that seems to be relieved when you eat certain foods. The mental symptoms can range from vague tension to acute restlessness, from nervousness to hyperactivity, and can include an inability to concentrate, insomnia, and even a marked change in personality. Food "addiction" can be so strong, and the withdrawal symptoms can be so severe, that they can result, literally, in an inability to function if the food is not eaten. For decades Theron G. Randolph, M.D., a clinical ecologist from Chicago, Illinois, who is a premier investigator in the field of bioecology, and his colleagues throughout the United States have tested and retested patients, and proved time and time again that food allergy and food addiction are often at the root of chronic compulsive overeating and obesity.

THE ALCOHOLISM CONNECTION

Are you a recovering alcoholic? Dr. Randolph discovered a link between alcoholism and an addictive form of food allergy.[2] In many cases he found compulsive drinking was a physical disorder, not a mental or emotional problem. (As early as 1956, Dr. Randolph described this phenomenon in *The Quarterly Review of Alcoholism*.) By testing patients with the food components of their favorite alcoholic drinks, Dr. Randolph discovered that many alcoholics were suffering from severe food allergies—allergies that caused symptoms of severe anxiety, nervousness, and depression, etc. These allergic reactions were precisely the same reactions that the compulsive drinker experienced when he or she did not have a drink and entered withdrawal. In one case study a recovering alcoholic who had not had a single drink in slightly over two years was tested by Dr. Randolph for possible food allergy. Dr. Randolph placed the patient on a program that for three days eliminated malt, wheat, and rye—the major ingredients in his patient's favorite drink—from his daily diet. During that three-day period, the compulsive drinker experienced withdrawal symptoms that he felt were completely incapacitating. Two days after the symptoms abated, Dr. Randolph gave his patient a test meal consisting solely of wheat products. Shortly thereafter, the patient again experienced a reaction that was "indistinguishable from the morning-after syndromes he had associated with his past drinking."[3] Clearly the patient had been consuming through food the substances that had been missing as a result of his two years of abstinance from alcoholic beverages. Obviously, the ethyl alcohol that was in his favorite drink was not the main addiction. (Because they recognize the link between alcoholism and food addiction, many alcoholism recovery centers recommend that the alcoholic carry something sweet around at all times to eat if the urge to drink surfaces.)

Although no one quite understands why people go through withdrawal (also known as hangovers, in the case of the alcoholic), professionals define the condition as existing while the body tries to cleanse itself of whatever is causing the reactions—be it food ingredient and/or chemical additive. By relying on an alternative source to obtain the substances he was addicted to in his drinks, the alcoholic postpones a thorough cleansing. Every time the level of specific food ingredients in his system drops below a certain point, his symptoms (anxiety, nervousness, depression, etc.) become more pronounced . . . and he eats again.

This substitution is not conscious. Only through happenstance does he find that corn, barley (malt), rye, and yeast (all of which are found in bourbon, for example) make him feel better . . . or the rye, wheat, potato yeast, possibly beet sugar, and cane syrup (all of which are present in domestic vodka) make him feel as terrific as a sip of his old favorite drink; although without the ethyl alcohol ingredient, he does not get inebriated.

Predictably, as in any addiction, tolerance levels change. As a consequence, he begins to eat more and more of these foods, just as during his alcoholic days he drank ever-increasing amounts of his favorite alcoholic beverage. He relieves his symptoms by filling up on a variety of foodstuffs, from bread, cake, and candy, to pizza, spaghetti, pies, and crackers—all of which contain food ingredients found in alcoholic beverages, and all of which are highly caloric. (More about increased tolerance and food addiction, shortly.)

Because without the presence of alcohol, absorption of materials in the upper intestinal tract is relatively slow, the recovering alcoholic does not get as immediate a sense of relief when he or she eats, rather than drinks, these foods. He or she does, however, definitely get a feeling of improved well-being as soon as the food is digested . . . and gains enormous weight in the process, as the addiction grows.

Of course, food allergy is not limited to people who were alcoholics. Nor does every food addict become overweight. Some people are allergic and addicted to low calorie foods, such as cauliflower or string beans, while other people have the bad luck to be allergic and addicted to very highly caloric foods like wheat, rice, red meat, and milk products. The former can eat in massive quantities, if they want to, and not gain weight, while the latter can barely squeeze into a chair with arms on it! *Invariably, however, the food to which a person is addicted is called a favorite food.*

Although researchers in the field of bioecology have discovered that repetition of the same foods over and over again can cause allergies to develop, bioecologists are not exactly certain why a form of food allergy that results in addiction exists. They are certain, however, that food addiction is real, as are the obese people who should know that there is something terribly wrong when they go to great lengths to obtain their favorite food. Addicted people have learned that without a portion of their favorite food—no substitute is acceptable—they are going to lose their feeling of well-being. They cannot endure the unpleasant physical and mental consequences of being deprived of their favorite (addictive) food even overnight. So, after slogging to and from the store, the "foodaholic" breaks open the package containing his favorite food. A swallow or two and, *voila!*, his head clears, he becomes charming and "normal" again. Suddenly he has a great deal of energy or, at last, he can sleep easily.

ARE YOU ADDICTED TO FOOD?

Are you a food-addicted person? If you answer "yes" to *any* of the following questions, the chances are very good indeed that food addiction is at the root of your problem. If your response is "no" to *all* of the questions, then you may probably rule out food addiction as a major factor in your weight gain.

	YES	NO
1. Do you experience headache, fatigue, weakness, depression, unreasonable irritability, etc., if you are late for or miss a meal?	___	___
2. Do you get relief from those discomforts if you eat?	___	___
3. Is supper incomplete if you do not have a specific food with it every single night?	___	___
4. Do you go on eating binges or food jags?	___	___
5. Do you keep your favorite candy in your pocket or purse, and munch on pieces of candy all day long?	___	___
6. Do you cover everything that can possibly take it with ketchup or mustard? Or relish? Or vinegar?	___	___
7. Do you have to make certain that you have a particular food or perhaps something sweet in the house all the time? Are you afraid to run out of it?	___	___
8. Do you have trouble facing the day without a doughnut or two, or without some particular food or beverage in the morning?	___	___
9. Do you have to eat bread, drink milk or coffee, or have some special food or beverage every day for lunch or at dinner time or as a snack between meals or late at night?	___	___
10. Do you have an almost insatiable craving for pizza, pancakes, cookies, cake, pretzels, spaghetti, or macaroni?	___	___
11. Do you have to eat a huge dish of ice cream or something else before you go to bed in order to sleep well?	___	___

ARE YOU ADDICTED TO FOOD?

	YES	NO
12. Do you keep a snack on your night stand ready for that middle-of-the-night hunger?	____	____
13. Do you insist on eating potatoes or corn in some form at every meal?	____	____
14. Do you feel there are some foods you could not live without?	____	____
15. Do you find it impossible to stick to a diet?	____	____
16. Do you admit to being a "junk food junky"?	____	____
17. Do you hide food in different places so you can always get at it?	____	____
18. Do you keep some food in your desk at work?	____	____
19. Do you still need to eat because you don't feel right even though a diet pill has completely eliminated your appetite?	____	____
20. Do you find, if you are a recovering alcoholic, that you now crave certain foods, rather than specific alcoholic drinks?	____	____

Source: Adapted from *Dr. Mandell's 5-Day Allergy Relief System,* by Marshall Mandell and Lynne Waller Scanlon.

All his symptoms of withdrawal subside . . . temporarily. He has had his "fix."

Also, as in any addiction, whether to drugs, or the chemicals and tobacco in cigarettes, there is an inevitable progression. What formerly could be satisfied by a snack in the evening begins to require a midday "fix" as well. Inevitably, not only do the number of "fixes" per day escalate, but the portion size increases as well. Eventually, you cannot complete your work day satisfactorily because mental and physical symptoms are interfering with your ability to perform your job. You cannot concentrate. You are terribly fatigued. Suddenly, your pockets are bursting with your "favorite" food and you *never* want to be without it. In fact, you now realize you *cannot* be without it. Your favorite snack is the only thing that makes you feel you can function. Between-meal eating becomes compellingly important to the addicted overeater, as are snacks just before bedtime in order to make it through the night without withdrawal symptoms. Ultimately, the severity of the problem makes it impossible to control eating, even though, rationally, you know you should not eat in such large amounts, or so frequently. Unfortunately, despite a very sincere desire to be healthy, slim and trim, you haven't got a chance unless you can break the addiction.

Did you answer "yes" to any of the questions on page 75? If so, then you should follow one of the three programs outlined later in this chapter in order to break the addiction before proceeding on to The 21st Century Diet. Once you have ended your addiction, you will discover that it is amazingly easy to follow The 21st Century Diet and lose weight . . . *and keep it off forever.*

Breaking Food Addiction

Breaking food addiction is actually not that difficult. There are three ways to go about it: the Food Elimination Method, the Rinkle Mono-Diet Method, and the Food Abstention Method. The first involves eliminating from your diet those high-risk foods that you would characterize as your "favorites" and that you habitually eat, and foods that tend to relieve any mental or physical complaints you might have; the second involves eating only *one* food at each meal; and the third involves a temporary abstention from all foods.

You are being given three choices because only you know the strength of your willpower and your ability to deny yourself. If you are fighting a slight weight problem, you are in a different category from the person who has now lost all control over food addiction and whose weight has soared to unmanageable levels that might include hundreds of extra pounds. Whether you have a twenty pound problem or a two hundred pound problem, if you answered "yes" to any of the questions in the beginning of this chapter, you suffer from food addiction to one degree or another.

All three methods work, although the first, the Food Elimination Method, may not be as effective as the other two techniques because it relies entirely on your ability to identify *all* the foods to which you are addicted and then avoid them religiously. Since food addiction may easily involve more than one food, it may be very difficult to isolate specific foods. Also, because food addiction is just that—an addiction—there is a tendency to rationalize not giving up a certain food. If you decide to try the Food Elimination Method but your addictions prove too strong, transfer to the Rinkle Mono-Diet Method and eat only the prescribed foods, or follow the Food Abstention Method and do not eat at all. All three plans take *four* days to complete.

Eleven People Who Can Help You

The following list of physicians should be helpful to those people on The 21st Century Diet who do not want to attempt to break food addiction on their own. Indeed, if you have ever been hospitalized for a life-threatening allergic reaction (asthma, for example), you should contact one of the people listed below, and place yourself under their supervision. If one of their offices is not conveniently located near you, a member of their staff should be able to recommend someone in your area who can help.

BIOECOLOGISTS IN THE UNITED STATES

John W. Argabrite, M.D.
First National Bank Building
P.O. Box 258
Watertown, SD 57201

Clifton R. Brooks, M.D.,
    M.P.H.
17400 W. Irvine Boulevard
Tustin, CA 92680

Thurman M. Bullock, Jr., M.D.
Murray F. Carrol, M.D.
722 N. Brown Street
Chadbourn, NC 28431

Kendal A. Gerdes, M.D.
Presbyterian Hospital
1719 East 19th Avenue
Denver, CO 80218

Harris Hosen, M.D.
2649 Proctor Street
Port Arthur, TX 77640

Verne A. Jackson, D.O.
1825 Maple Street
Forest Grove, OR 97116

Joseph T. Morgan, M.D.
Bay Clinic
1750 Thompson Road
Coos Bay, OR 97420

Dale W. Peters, M.D.
3201 East Second
Wichita, KS 67208

Theron G. Randolph, M.D.
505 North Lake Shore Dr.
Chicago, IL 60611

William J. Rea, M.D.
Suite 240
8345 Walnut Hill Lane
Dallas, TX 75231

If you have elected to try an "at home" method to break food addiction, begin by isolating potential problem foods in a preliminary step.

PRELIMINARY STEP

Since you are overweight, many of the foods to which you are addicted are going to be high calorie foods. However, food addiction is not limited to fattening foods, so do not be surprised if a few low calorie items enter the picture, too. No matter which plan you choose, first fill in the section below with your favorite foods, those foods you have every day, and those foods that make you feel physically or mentally better after you eat them. In doing so, you will get an accurate picture of the foods that may be causing your problem.

FOODS TO WHICH YOU MAY BE ADDICTED

	FAVORITE FOODS	FOODS EATEN EVERY DAY	SYMPTOM-ALLEVIATING FOODS
1.			
2.			
3.			
4.			
5.			
6.			
7.			
8.			
9.			
10.			

Now look at your list. Any food that appears should be implicated as a potential "addictive" food. Also, as stated earlier in this chapter, it has been proved by Dr. Theron Randolph that compulsive drinkers are often addicted to the food ingredients in their favorite drinks, not the ethyl alcohol component. If you have given up alcoholic beverages and find that you crave specific foods, take a look at the list below. Specifically, the following foods are commonly found in wine, beer, rum, whiskey, and vodka. Do not be surprised if some of them appear on your list:

Grape Wine: raisins or grapes, beets or beet sugar, brewer's yeast, cane sugar, corn, eggs (used in clearing some wines)
Beer: brown rice, barley, malt, brewer's yeast, corn
Rum: cane sugar, brewer's yeast
Whiskey and Vodka: white potato, rye, corn, wheat, barley

As you research the caloric content of your favorite foods, you are going to begin to see that items like grain, sugar, red meat, milk products (cheeses, butter, whole milk), nuts, and some beans make your list repeatedly. After all, these are the foods that contain the most calories. People addicted to carrots don't suffer the same weight consequences as people addicted to peanuts; one-half a cup of chopped carrots contains approximately 42 calories, whereas a handful of peanuts has 585 calories. A modest dish of sliced pears in heavy syrup is 76 calories, but a small bowl of shredded wheat is 363 calories.

THE FOOD ELIMINATION METHOD

In order to follow the Food Elimination Method, you must now eliminate from your diet *all* those foods that made your list. Obviously, since the favorite foods of foodaholics dominate their daily menus, you are going to experience a radical change in your meals. Glance at The Biological Classification of Foods in Chapter Three for some suggestions in planning your new regimen. Select foods that are from separate families. Try to keep your meals simple and straightforward: broiled chicken, steamed peas and carrots, or steamed shrimp, broccoli and mushrooms, for instance.

In order for the Food Elimination Method to work successfully, you are going to have to get into the habit of reading labels. If, for example, wheat is on your "forbidden foods" list, then you should be aware that just to avoid wheat-based breads and the more obvious wheat sources will not guarantee that you won't encounter wheat hidden in some other food items. To give you an indication of the type of investigative process involved, the following is a partial listing of foods that you might not suspect contain wheat, sugar, or milk, but may, depending upon whether you have had a hand in determining the ingredients or whether the ingredients have been chosen by the company producing the product.

WHEAT	SUGAR	MILK
Alcoholic beverages	Alcoholic beverages	Bologna
Bologna	Canned fruits	Doughnuts
Bouillon	Canned vegetables	Gravies
Candy	Catsup	Hamburgers
Farina	Cereals	Meatloaf
Ice cream	Gum	Sauces
Liverwurst	Jarred horseradish	Sausages
Pudding	Mayonnaise	Sherbet
Soups	Salad dressings	Soups
Vitamin E	Sausages	
	Soy sauce	
	Steak sauce	
	Toothpaste	
	Yogurt	

During the course of the Food Elimination Method, if you feel your withdrawal symptoms surfacing, take Alka Seltzer Gold (not the regular, blue-wrapped Alka Seltzer; it contains aspirin). Take two tablets in two eight-ounce glasses of water and within a matter of minutes (twenty at the most) your symptoms will subside. *Do not take more frequently than recommended on the package.* The alkaline salts contained in Alka Seltzer Gold neutralize and stop allergic withdrawal symptoms as the salts return your body chemistry to normal. You can also mix your own salts by combining two level tablespoons of baking soda with one level tablespoon of potassium bicarbonate in a four- to six-ounce container. Shake until mixed well. Stir one-half teaspoon of the mixture into each of two large glasses of water. *Consult your doctor if you have heart, kidney disease, high blood pressure, or must restrict your sodium intake for* ANY *reason before you take the alkaline salts remedy.*

You may lose a great deal of weight on the first few days of the Food Elimination method. Allergic people often experience bloating in the face, hands, and feet. During an allergic reaction, the thin-walled capillary blood vessels are temporarily altered, allowing fluids to escape from your blood stream into the surrounding tissue. As you eliminate the foods that are causing this "allergic edema," you may find that as much as five to ten pounds of fluid will be eliminated. Don't worry. This fluid loss is often the first sign that you are breaking the grip of addiction.

After four days your system will have begun to clean out the food residues in your digestive tract. With the help of an occasional laxative over these four days, you can speed the process up. If not having your favorite foods for that length of time seems terribly self-sacrificing, know that after the four-day period, you won't crave them any more strongly than you crave a food that didn't make your list. After completing the Elimination Method, proceed to The 21st Century Diet.

THE RINKLE MONO-DIET METHOD

Herbert Rinkle, M.D., a pioneer in the field of bioecology, developed the Rinkle Mono-Diet Method to help his patients determine foods causing their allergic symptoms and, ultimately, as a means to eliminate the symptoms. It was Dr. Rinkle who discovered that patients who did not encounter the same food item more frequently than once in four days were immune from two out of three types of food allergy: cyclical and addictive. This "rotation" of foods to which the patient was allergic—foods referred to as "offenders" by allergists—lifted the "allergic burden" placed on extremely food-sensitive people.

Since it is now known that eating the same foods every day can cause you to develop allergic reactions to those foods, by staggering your exposure to all foods (those to which you are allergic as well as those foods to which you are not), you derive two benefits: you eliminate the mental and physical symptoms associated with cyclical and addictive food allergies, and you protect yourself from developing new food allergies.

If you have decided to use the Rinkle Mono-Diet Method to break your food addiction, just follow the simple one-food-at-a-time menu below for four days, then proceed to The 21st Century Diet.

RINKLE MONO-DIET METHOD

Directions: Eat as large a portion as you would like at each meal. Separate the meals by at least three hours. Preferably, eat foods that are as close to natural as possible so that you can eliminate residues from pesticides, insecticides, herbicides, food colorings, and preservatives, to which you may also be allergic. The only liquid you should have is spring water, lots of it. If you have any difficulty with cravings or mental and physical symptoms, immediately drink two large glasses of spring water that contain one tablet each of Alka Seltzer Gold (not the blue-wrapped, regular Alka Seltzer, which contains aspirin). Your symptoms will subside within a matter of minutes. *If, however, you have kidney or heart disease, high blood pressure or must restrict sodium intake for ANY reason, consult your doctor before taking the alkaline salts remedy.*

The four-day meal plan below is divided into specific "families of foods" that are based on biological classifications as explained in detail in Chapter Three. No one family appears more than once, thus ensuring Dr. Rinkle's rotation method.

	MEAL #1	MEAL #2	MEAL #3	MEAL #4
Day #1	*Rose Family* apples or pears	*Gourd Family* squash	*Bovine Family* lamb or beef	*Grass Family* rice or corn
Day #2	*Banana Family* bananas	*Cashew Family* cashews or pistachios	*Pheasant Family* chicken or eggs	*Goosefoot Family* beets or spinach
Day #3	*Swine Family* bacon or pork	*Carrot Family* carrots	*Turkey Family* turkey	*Grape Family* grapes or raisins
Day #4	*Rue Family* grapefruit or oranges	*Legume Family* lima beans or string beans	*Mackerel Family* albacore or tuna	*Potato Family* potatoes or tomatoes

At the end of the four-day period on the Rinkle Mono-Diet Method, you will find your "allergic burden" lifted and your food addictions broken. You should feel better than you have felt in years, cravings should have abated, and, if you suffered from water retention in your face, hands, or feet, you will find that this, too, has disappeared, as have the five to ten pounds that "allergic edema" can represent.

Now you are ready for The 21st Century Diet, which will continue the rotation process, but incorporate more food choices and limit calories.

THE FOOD ABSTENTION METHOD

Sometimes it is easier not to eat at all, instead of selecting and eliminating certain foods. You should always, however, consult your doctor before undertaking a fast. If, in his or her opinion, a fast is all right for you, go ahead. Simply stop eating and, since tap water often contains chemicals, start drinking large quantities of spring water instead. Every time you crave food, go over to the refrigerator and pour yourself another glass of water. Keep sipping . . . for about four days.

Since symptoms of withdrawal will begin shortly after you miss the first portion of the food to which you are addicted, the best time to begin the Food Abstention Method is when you have several days to devote to it and when you will not be inconvenienced by the mental and physical symptoms associated with withdrawal. Even though there is a remedy, discussed below, to lessen these symptoms, you really do not want to be in a situation where you have to perform at your best during a period when you are undergoing a bodywide biochemical upheaval.

The following is a list of tips to get you started and to give you some insight into what to expect if abstaining from all food is your preferred choice:

● The night before you begin, take a mild laxative, and repeat every other day for the duration of the plan if you feel constipated or listless. (Use milk of magnesia—unflavored—or magnesium citrate.) This cleans out food residues in your digestive tract, including those to which you are allergic and addicted. After all, the digestive tract—a tube more than forty feet long from mouth to anus—is the site of the thermal, mechanical, and chemical processing of foods you eat. Once these foods are broken down into small enough particles, they are absorbed through the "inner skin" of the intestinal wall and into your body.

- Another option is to give yourself periodic spring water enemas as an aid to thorough cleansing of your intestional tract, of which the lower bowel is the final section. Use a pint of spring water that has adjusted to room temperature; add one level teaspoon of baking soda or sea salt.

- Do not make the mistake of running short on spring water. On the first day in particular, you will find that you make constant trips to the refrigerator. This is the result of combination of the "habit" of constantly nibbling and the "obsession" with food because you are addicted. If you run out of spring water, you will be tempted to drink tap water. Don't do it! Not just any water is acceptable; spring water is free of the chemicals commonly found in tap water, and you want to "purify" your system as thoroughly as possible. Also, bear in mind that the frequency of trips to the refrigerator will lessen as time passes, although it will certainly seem as if you always have a glass of spring water in your hand on the first day! By the second day, you will be tapering off as you break not only the habit of improper eating, but your addiction as well.

- Remember, *you will feel worse before you feel better.* However you will also find that each flare-up of symptoms will be less severe than the last, until you are symptom-free. Any time you have a resurgence of withdrawal symptoms, take an Alka Seltzer Gold (not the regular, blue-wrapped Alka Seltzer, which contains aspirin) as instructed on page 81. *However, if you have heart or kidney disease, high blood pressure, or must restrict sodium intake for any reason, check with your doctor before taking alkaline salts in any form.*

- Be prepared for rapid weight loss, up to five to ten pounds within the first day or two. Don't worry. Rapid weight loss on the first day or two is simply an indication that "allergic edema" is also one of your problems. As soon as you stop eating the foods that are causing the problem, the problem subsides. Don't expect many "true" pounds to come off during these four days. In fact, as you may recall from a previous chapter, your metabolic rate will slow down dramatically over these four days because of an instinctive mechanism that comes into play to help you survive famine. Although you may lose a fraction of a pound or two in fat, it will be the actual 21st Century Diet that will be responsible for successful dieting.

- Bioecologists have also found that high blood pressure can be an allergic response to foods. If you have high blood pressure, do not be surprised if your blood pressure drops when you stop eating, and even goes down to what is considered "normal limits." Check and recheck your blood pressure. Keep your doctor informed of your results. It is just possible that you could obtain information that indicates your "essential" hypertension is actually an allergic reaction.

- You may get chills or begin to perspire. Ride out these symptoms, too. They will pass. Just keep sipping!

- Be prepared for some occasional weakness. If it occurs, try an enema or some alkaline salts. Despite all the spring water, you may also be a little dehydrated, so keep sipping. The weakness will pass. Give it some time.

- Expect a little lethargy. Your metabolic rate will be telling you to slow down and preserve your energy reserves.

- Avoid vitamin and mineral supplements for this four-day period. On an empty stomach, vitamins and minerals can nauseate you or give you heartburn.

- Do not take nonessential medication, including aspirin. If you are not feeling well, remember that this is only a four-day ordeal—not your entire life. Take only those medications prescribed by your doctor, and be sure to mention that you are fasting, in case he or she wants to alter your medication accordingly. Ideally, you should not take any drugs or medications, prescription or nonprescription, over the four-day period. Check with your doctor and ask if you may eliminate all your drugs. After all, you are trying to cleanse your system totally.

- Try not to smoke. Even though you think that giving up food for four days is difficult enough, now might be the time to give up cigarettes, also. A number of people using this technique have reported that it was much less of a trial to forego cigarettes during the period they did not eat than it was at any other time in their lives. Cigarettes are replete with chemicals, literally hundreds, that impart flavor or that had a role in seeing that the tobacco plant reached maturity and did not succumb to parasites. Even the paper that tobacco is wrapped in has chemical residues. Obviously, the decision is yours, but remember, you are trying to create an environment within your body that is food-free . . . and as chemical-free as possible.

• Use sea salt or baking soda when you brush your teeth. Either one does an excellent job. Toothpaste and mouthwash have chemicals in them that, like food, will be absorbed through your intestinal tract.

Not eating is really easier than it sounds. It might seem like great deprivation, particularly to the foodaholic, but you will be surprised at how easy it becomes. Franz Kafka wrote a wonderful short story called "A Hunger Artist" in which a man made his living by specializing in public fasting for a living. He would draw great crowds to his cage at the circus or in the town square. Amazed people marveled at his ability to give up food for weeks at a time. What they did not know, and what he mused about, was how very easy his chosen career was. As anyone who has fasted will tell you, after the first day or two, fasting becomes almost effortless.

At the end of the first day, as your body makes a transition from expecting incoming food to utilizing stored supplies, all hunger pangs cease. (Yes, your metabolism will slow down too, but don't worry about it. Four consecutive days without food will not cause the type of diet-resistant difficulties associated with weight loss that chronic starving and binging produce. And if you are already guilty of overeating followed by undereating, your metabolism is already disrupted, and you will not make the situation any worse.) By the time four days have passed, you will find all cravings have subsided, too, as have all the symptoms associated with food addiction withdrawal. For perhaps the first time in your life, you will not be handicapped by the debilitating consequences of food addiction.

Upon starting the actual 21st Century Diet, you may find you do not have much of an appetite. Just eat what you can for the first day or two. After that your capacity for food will increase, and you will be back to normal. Also, bear in mind that bioecologists have found that after avoiding foods that may have caused you allergic problems in the past (headache, compulsive eating, irritability, bloating), you may be supersensitive to them now. If you know a food on The 21st Century Diet is a potential problem food, or discover that a specific meal causes you allergic symptoms, simply substitute appropriate foods from the selections you will find available in each diet plan (800 calories, 1200 calories, or 1600 calories), and continue the diet.

If you are a food-addicted person, you must conquer the addiction *before* you start the actual 21st Century Diet. Although The 21st Century Diet recognizes the phenomenon of food addiction and is designed to help prevent you from perpetuating your addiction or developing new addictions (a serious problem for the person with a predisposition to food addiction), you must recognize your problem and dispense with it. Since food addiction—not a psychological problem or a disorder of the will—has been the major cause of your inability to sustain a diet, break the addiction first, then move on to The 21st Century Diet.

Whichever method you have chosen to break your food addiction, once you have completed four days, you should be well on your way to successful dieting with The 21st Century Diet.

NOTES

1. Theron G. Randolph, M.D., and Ralph W. Moss, Ph.D., *An Alternative Approach to Allergies* (New York: Lippincott & Crowell, 1980), p. 17.
2. Ibid., pp. 109–116.
3. Marshall Mandell, M.D., and Lynne Waller Scanlon, *Dr. Mandell's 5-Day Allergy Relief System* (New York: T.Y. Crowell, 1979), p. 118.

8

Taking the Obsession out of Dieting

FACT: You cannot keep weight off simply by counting and being obsessed about calories.

FACT: You *must* choose from among three plans to ensure consistent calorie reduction and maintenance.

FACT: You do not have to exercise to lose weight, but doing so increases your metabolic rate and can account for as much as 52 pounds a year.

FACT: You can derive more benefits if you exercise during the afternoon and early evening.

FACT: Your body ages not from overeating, but from disuse.

Calories: Avoid 'em, Burn 'em, and Reinforce Their Departure

For many people dieting has been a way of life—a continuous obsession that pervades every day . . . and every meal . . . and every conversation. Yet, your whole life should not revolve around an obsessive desire to lose weight or keep it off. Spending hours of mental energy constantly fretting about gaining a pound or losing a pound or maintaining a desired weight level or when your next meal or snack will be takes much too much valuable time and energy away from other more interesting pursuits. Counting calories, arranging meals, and continually thinking about food not only waste time and energy, but have proven unsuccessful in permanently reducing weight. Successful dieting constitutes a release from the constant, every day, every meal concern that permeates the dieter's life, and develops the ability virtually to forget about weight and banish food worries to the recesses of your mind. To lose sufficient weight and lose your anxiety about your weight forever, you must consciously reorganize your approach to weight loss and avail yourself of techniques, other than actually counting your calories, that have proved successful adjuncts to dieting.

How do you begin? Take a look at your professed goals for dieting and your overall weight reduction strategy to attain those goals.

Are Your Personal Goals Sufficient Motivation?

You are about to begin a diet, either for the first time or for what seems like the hundredth time. You may say, "I'm dieting to lose weight," but that is really only part of the story. Chances are, you are dieting to look more attractive, to improve your health, or to enhance your physical capabilities—the three reasons most cited by dieters as the motivating force behind cutting calories. Unfortunately, studies have shown that the first, second, and third reasons mentioned above—without bringing other factors into play—are not sufficient to guarantee that you will lose the amount of weight you desire, or that you will keep the weight off. In fact, the odds are against you.

LOSING WEIGHT TO IMPROVE HEALTH

Rarely is a person successful at dieting when the only motivation for losing weight is strictly to improve the quality of his or her health. Even though being overweight is *always* an indication of impaired health, knowledge of this does not, by itself, initiate change effectively, nor can it assure sustained change. Despite all the evidence that directly links adult-onset diabetes, shortness of breath, chronic fatigue, increased blood pressure, back and joint pain, bloating, and susceptibility to infection to being seriously overweight, a simple desire to diet for improved health has proved to be insufficient for sustaining the resolve of the majority of dieters—other than those already seriously ill with a weight-related ailment—

in their weight reduction efforts. Most dieters in this category simply lose interst in their diet after a short while and quickly resume their old eating patterns.

LOSING WEIGHT TO LOOK MORE ATTRACTIVE

In other cases, people begin monitoring their caloric intake in order to improve their physical appearance. If you readily admit to wanting to improve your silhouette, chances are, studies have shown, you are female. (Although men diet for the same reason, they appear to be more reluctant to admit that sheer vanity is at the core of their motivation!) Because of the emphasis on thinness in the fashion world, many women want to see a lean silhouette reflected back in the mirror. Unfortunately, anyone whose sole motivation to count calories is to improve looks often succeeds in taking some weight off, but rarely succeeds in keeping it off. The number of repeat dieters attests to this fact.

LOSING WEIGHT TO BE MORE AGILE

Some people diet to improve sense of balance and agility. Indeed, men more often than women, diet to improve physical prowess. With additional poundage, men find that their bellies get in the way hanging over the waistline of their pants, or their thighs rub together when they walk. Overweight men feel (and are) clumsy and want to do something about their awkwardness. Like the desire to improve health or appearance, the motivation to watch caloric intake primarily for improved agility has proved, time and time again, unable to guarantee success.

The Secret to Making The 21st Century Diet Your Last Diet Effort

The Fun Factor: In a study of volunteers who claimed to be dieting strictly for improved health, it was found that the only successful participants—those who actually completed the study—were people who discovered that they could continue to monitor their caloric intake *because they grew to enjoy and derive personal pleasure from some of the study's secondary elements,* even if they loathed actually limiting their food intake. The study concluded that the dieters would not have continued to diet without the fun factor, even though the participants continually lost weight and/or knew they were improving their health as the study progressed.[1] What constituted "fun" and provided encouragement varied from person to person, but one element seemed uniformly present: the "fun" aspect eventually superseded the "desire" to lose weight as the main weight loss motivation. For some of the successful dieters it was the newfound friendships and sense of camaraderie among fellow participants that encouraged them and kept them dieting. For others it was the thrill of discovering an ability to perform an activity or a sport in which they were forced, in a sense, to participate by the study. It was a combination of factors that bolstered and reinforced the commitment to continue to limit calories—factors that had little to do with a longing to become more physically attractive, or to attain better health, or to become able to tighten a belt another notch or two. The study dropouts, on the other hand, had failed to find *any* of the aspects of the study, including calorie counting, sufficiently enjoyable to enable them to summon the motivation to continue dieting, even though they had eagerly volunteered at the study's onset.

Indeed, the dieter deludes him or herself by thinking that the simple "desire" to lose weight, for whatever reason, is sufficient to guarantee lasting results. In those instances when weight loss was achieved, the victory was, more often than not, temporary. Moreover, it was only accomplished by dint of "superhuman" and "obsessive" effort—both unnecessary and self-defeating ingredients in the truly successful diet.

Why You Keep Losing the Same Old Pounds

Dieting should be merely one component of a grand scheme in which you attack the problem of weight control from a variety of directions. Only by a multifront attack will you be able to stay slim and trim in the future without any need to repeat the kind of effort and will power necessary to reach your desired weight. Calorie counting is not enough.

Even though dieters can receive reinforcement by experiencing actual weight loss, that encouragement has proved not to be sufficient to maintain the diet. This is why so many dieters take the same few pounds off, then quit. Rarely do dieters reach their expressed goals. Even more rarely do they maintain that weight goal. Of course, if you want to be like the typical repeat dieter and lose an average of sixteen pounds *each time you diet,* and do not mind monthly or annual struggles with the same poundage, then you can simply resign yourself to periodic obsession with a diet.

The 21st Century Diet is designed to help you create an approach to weight loss that makes shedding pounds an inevitable by-product of activities (including a choice of physical and/or emotional support systems) that you find enjoyable. By offering the kind of integrated approach that encourages and reinforces dieting, by taking the primary focus off the fixation with food, per se, and by including a unique menu design, The 21st Century Diet virtually guarantees that you will have the proper blend of elements that will turn you from a perpetual dieter into a successful dieter.

One of the keys to the success of The 21st Century Diet is that you will create an atmosphere that is both pleasurable and effective. Your initial approach will be carefully planned, and will require a few decisions and some thought on your part. However, the results of The 21st Century Diet multifaceted approach will quickly be apparent, and you will be able to continue with enthusiasm until you reach your desired weight goal. Essentially, you have three approaches from which to choose to complete your diet plan. Although often one is enough, ideally, you should try the tripartite approach.

OPTION #1—REDUCING YOUR ENERGY CRISIS

Although half of the people in America get no vigorous exercise at all,[2] exercise is one of the best ways to take weight off. The fringe benefits are enormous and immediate. In fact, you would not have to diet at all to lose weight if you increased your amount of exercise sufficiently. Howard F. Hunt, chairman of the physical education department at the University of California, San Diego, speaking at an annual food editors conference, debunked the myth that exercise burns calories off too slowly. Hunt said, "The real benefit of exercise is that it can lead to a higher metabolic rate for two to ten hours afterwards. That can account for as much as fifty-two pounds a year."[3] After all, extra weight is the result of energy intake (calories in food) exceeding energy depletion (calories burned). You do not see any marathoners carrying extra weight.

Of course, there are people who simply will not exercise. They assume that there is no way that they are going to get up an hour before work or find the time in the evening to jog around town. If you are one of those, bear in mind what Molly Salazar, new mother and wife of Alberto Salazar (three-time winner of the New York Marathon), said about her attitude toward running. "It wasn't love at first try. At first I hated it. I stayed because my coach made it interesting and because I enjoyed the girls on the team."[4] (The fun factor!) You don't have to exercise an hour a day to reap the benefits. Even a little helps. If you find a walk to the local general store out of the question, chances are that your initiating a vigorous exercise program is even more unlikely. Often, the more sedentary (and overweight) you have become, the more difficult it is even to start to exercise, no matter how light that exercise is. If you become winded climbing a flight of stairs, you should start an exercise program gradually and take the time you need to build up to vigorous exercise. Another deterrent many out-of-shape people face is an embarrassment at being seen exercising in public. What they do not realize is that their "public" gives them enormous credit for actively doing something to get in shape. This favorable reaction occurs particularly in those people who are in shape now, but were once as out of shape as you are.

OPTION #2—GENTLE GROUP PRESSURE AND ENCOURAGEMENT

Two (or more) can do it better than one. Family members who are also overweight, friends who complain as bitterly as you do about constant dieting, professional groups, anyone who has a desire to lose weight but who has failed consistently, would be a good candidate for participating in a diet plan. It is much easier (and even might have the dimension of "fun") to diet on the buddy system, checking in with each other and encouraging friendly competition, than it is to go it alone. Plus, group participation has *proved* to be highly effective.

When you create or join a group you will make new friends and may even develop outside interests that will expand your horizons. Since everyone in the group is trying to lose excess weight, you have something in common to talk about right from the start. If you are hesitant about joining a group in which you do not know anyone, bring an overweight friend or relative along at least for the first meeting. If you don't have anyone to go with you, call ahead and ask if you could arrange to travel over to the meeting with a member or be met at the door. People in these groups are usually very nice, very sympathetic, and very understanding . . . and very goal-oriented, too. Remember, it is the meetings themselves that lend impetus to continuing on the weight loss program, not the actual diet. Even though participants may not have realized this "intellectually," weight loss is a continuing by-product of the meetings, which not only encourage members in their weight loss efforts, but also provide an avenue for developing new friendships and activities.

OPTION #3—THE TRIPARTITE APPROACH

Either one of the above options will help ensure that you will succeed, almost despite yourself, on your diet plan. However, the ideal program incorporates a tripartite combination of exercise,

APPROACHES TO WEIGHT LOSS

OPTION	Prospects for Success			
	DISMAL	GOOD	BETTER	BEST
Count calories	x			
Forced exercise	x			
Enjoyable exercise	xxxxxxxxxxxxxxxxxxxx			
Encouragement group	xxxxxxxxxxxxxxxxxxxx			
Count calories *and* enjoyable exercise		xxxxxxxxxxxxxxxxxxxxxxxxxxxxxx		
Count calories *and* group support		xxxxxxxxxxxxxxxxxxxxxxxxxxxxxx		
Count calories *and* enjoyable exercise *and* group support		xxxxxxxxxxxxxxxxxxxxxxxxxxxxxxxxxxxxxxxxx		

group support, and calorie counting that you follow until you reach your weight loss goal and are able to maintain that reduction without much concern for calories. Exercise and the friendships derived from group support will continue as part of your new lifestyle even after you have reached your weight goal.

Again, you do not have to participate in any one of the options. If you do not want to exercise, don't. If the thought of joining or creating a group seems beyond comprehension, don't. If the possibility of doing a little of both seems completely out of the question, don't. As long as you incorporate the general scheme of The 21st Century Diet (with its emphasis on the rotation of foods to lessen cravings and on consuming the preponderance of calories during the daytime hours to assure more efficient digestion of food) you will experience a drop in your weight. However, you will have to work much harder at it and much more diligently than your fellow dieters who, after a period of time, should be able to relegate active dieting and "obsession" with food to the past. Moreover, keeping those pounds you lost off will be more difficult for you.

If you think you might be able to make a few changes in your overall approach to dieting, answer the following questionnaire. It should enable you to narrow your interests (or possible interests) down, and give you a starting point. Consider the activities in which you have participated in the past, would like to try in the future, or could conceivably hold any interest for you at all. Bear in mind that for you to gain a pound you have to increase your food intake by 3500 calories, and to lose one pound you must deny your body 4000 calories that it is used to getting. There are two ways to accomplish the 4000 figure—cut calories and/or burn them. Either method will have a noticeable effect. Together, however, they make a combination punch.

OPTIONAL ATHLETIC ACTIVITIES

ACTIVITY	YES	NO	MAYBE
Badminton	----	----	----
Baseball			
hardball	----	----	----
softball	----	----	----
Basketball	----	----	----

OPTIONAL ATHLETIC ACTIVITIES

ACTIVITY	YES	NO	MAYBE
Bicycling	___	___	___
Bowling	___	___	___
Calisthenics	___	___	___
Canoeing	___	___	___
Dancing			
aerobic	___	___	___
ballroom	___	___	___
disco	___	___	___
jazzercize	___	___	___
Football	___	___	___
Gardening	___	___	___
Golf	___	___	___
Gymnastics	___	___	___
Handball	___	___	___
Hockey			
field	___	___	___
ice	___	___	___
Horseback riding	___	___	___
Jogging	___	___	___
Lacrosse	___	___	___
Racquet ball	___	___	___
Rowing	___	___	___
Rugby	___	___	___
Skating			
ice	___	___	___
roller	___	___	___
Skiing			
alpine	___	___	___
cross country	___	___	___
water	___	___	___
Soccer	___	___	___
Softball	___	___	___
Squash	___	___	___
Swimming	___	___	___
Table tennis	___	___	___
Volleyball	___	___	___
Walking	___	___	___
Windsurfing	___	___	___

The Best Time of Day to Exercise

Does it really matter at what time of day you exercise? Scientists say yes. Just as your circadian or daily body rhythms affect your waking and sleeping patterns (making you drowsy in the evening about the same time every night, and causing you to awaken at the same time every morning), so do rhythms influence your body temperature (rising to 98.6 degrees in the daytime and dropping at night by as much as 1.20 degrees); your sense of smell (food tastes better in the evening); your hearing (television sets are turned up and children are more easily tuned out in the evening hours); and your athletic ability. According to Dr. K. E. Klein at the Institute for Flight Medicine in Bad Godesberg, Germany, reaction time and complex motor performance are at their peak, on the average, between one o'clock in the afternoon and seven o'clock in the evening.[5]

Does this mean that you should not exercise except between those hours? No. Any exercise is better than no exercise, no matter what time during the day you choose to participate. What studies indicate however, is that if it is at all possible to schedule your exercise during the early afternoon or early evening, not only will you perform better and more easily, but you will make more rapid progress in your pursuit of a more toned, flexible body than if you exercise in the morning or late at night.

Also, bear in mind that *any* exercise increases metabolic rate—no matter what the time of day—and more and more evidence indicates that once turned up to a higher speed, metabolic rate tends to maintain an increased speed for up to half a day or more.[6] A brisk walk for twenty minutes after breakfast or supper (eating also increases metabolism for the digestive process) can result in your metabolism speeding along at a more rapid clip for the entire 24-hour day!

Exercise? *Moi?*

When you augment your approach to dieting with exercise, as a bonus you will tone up your muscles, replacing fat with firmness. Of course, if you are in very bad physical shape, and get winded, as mentioned previously, by something as simple as ascending a flight of steps, you are going to have to pace yourself carefully. Take a step at a time, figuratively. The following is a list of typical excuses that dieters use to talk themselves out of exercising while they follow a weight reduction diet:

1. *You will lose the weight first, then exercise.* Not a good idea. Weight loss is accelerated through exercise. And you will tone up, rather than be thin but sagging under your clothes. Your body has its own "appestat," a kind of control system that regulates and balances the amount of energy expended and the desire for caloric intake. Exercise actually takes the edge off appetite, as your body turns to its own stored reserves.

2. *You are just too busy to fit exercise into your schedule.* Too tired after work. Too busy before work. As difficult as it seems to work up the enthusiasm to stick to an exercise program and as easy as it is to talk yourself out of dragging yourself to the gym or pulling your "sweats" out of the drawer, once you participate long enough, you will discover that no excuse is a good excuse. From the moment you manage to get going, you will feel more energized. And at the end of the exercise, you will feel both psychologically better and physically renewed. Exercise stimulates the pituitary gland in the brain, which in turn produces high levels of beta endorphins that give you a natural "high" that helps you cope with physical and psychological stress . . . and helps keep your appetite level down. You will feel terrific after just a little exercise. Get up and get going!

3. *You feel too embarrassed to be seen by "your public" in your present condition.* You can check your local television listings to find a half-hour exercise class and work out in the privacy of your own house or apartment, or you can buy an exercise record. However, it is important to understand that many of the sleek joggers you see moving along country roads or down city streets at dawn or dusk were in questionable shape themselves at one time. The same holds true for men and women working out in organized exercise programs. The truth is that everyone has enormous respect for someone who is overweight and out of shape, but who is actively doing something about it. No one looks down on a person who is making

a concerted effort to shape up; particularly not the svelte athlete who knows the kind of effort involved. You will be given credit for finally getting started.

4. *You are not sure in which sport to participate.* Are you competitive, aggressive, self-motivated, introverted, or extroverted? Ask yourself whether you are a loner (by preference, rather than because you feel too fat to socialize) or a more gregarious type who enjoys interacting with others. If you would rather not have to talk to anyone while you concentrate on working out, try those sports that do not require more than one person: bicycling, jogging, walking, gardening, swimming, canoeing. But remember, group participation can be fun, and casual pressure from the group will encourage you to continue exercising. If you like hobnobbing, join a team sport. You do not have to be in great shape. Often, as in rugby, there are first, second, and third string teams—even the "old man's" squad for the over forty and winded set. Getting started is as easy as checking the telephone book Yellow Pages to see what is available in your area. Look under gymnasiums, health clubs, sports clubs. Give them a call and get details. Find out if they have special programs for people losing weight. You may be very surprised to see how many people are involved in a slimming program that involves initially mild exercise.

5. *You won't know anybody in any of the sports programs.* When you speak to the program organizers, mention the fact that you probably won't know a soul, and ask if there is any one person who will be introducing you. Don't worry; it is usually very easy to meet and talk to your fellow participants. Another alternative is to bring along a friend who is also interested in weight loss.

6. *You feel too old to participate.* Part of the aging process results in a thinning out of bones that makes them frail and subject to breaks. Some physicians feel that the preponderance of hip bone breaks experienced by the elderly may actually have resulted from a misstep that broke the bone *before* the elderly person hit the ground. You have 200 separate bones that protect your vulnerable inner parts, including the spinal cord, the brain, and the heart (actually itself a muscle). The main thing you have between you and the collapse of your skeleton or inner scaffolding is contractile muscle, with an

overlay of skin. Aging and collapse are more often the result of disuse than overuse, particularly among people over 65, the age group known to exercise less than any other. Humans, like plants, become weakened and frail with too much indoor life. Yet, exercise produces an increased, strengthened volume of muscle tissue that will enable you to function more efficiently and with more confidence. As a by-product, exercise causes biochemical changes that actually increase bone strength, helping to counteract the thinning process that is underway. Just as you would expose a plant to the outdoors very carefully, allowing it to "harden off" first by a little exposure to the elements each day, so should you proceed with caution if you are elderly. Start off slowly, walking as briskly as possible everyday. Join a senior citizens' exercise class. Work against the ravages of deteriorating diseases, like arthritis, which have proved to respond favorably to exercise. Do not fall into a vicious cycle of decreasing activity as a result of chronic pain or discomfort due to rickety bones. Build them up as best you can. The actual act of exercise will trigger opiumlike natural chemicals in your brain that will help relieve pain. There is pleasure in exercise. Avail yourself of it.

If you elect not to exercise, you *must* at least join a group of people who are working together to lose weight. Chances are you are an old hand at dieting. There is a reason you have kept all those different sized clothes, and it is because no diet has yet worked for you permanently. The 21st Century Diet research has proved you cannot lose weight and expect to keep it off without help, or you would not be contemplating another diet now! You *must* get reinforcement. If you do not want to join a group at your local YMCA or YWCA, or any of the health clubs or clinics that specialize in weight loss, then enlist the aid of overweight friends. Organize. They need group support also. Plan weekly meetings to discuss weight loss progress. As part of the weekly meeting, plan excursions to museums and nature trails. Add a new dimension to your life besides the diet and reap some extra benefits from intellectual stimulation. Participate in group activities involving physical exertion that will lop a few calories off, if only on the day you and your group tour a museum or amble along a path. Look around you, in your immediate family, on your street, in your church or synagogue, at your club or school, for the support and fun you need to diet effectively.

If you elect to join a health club, choose one that takes exercise seriously. The idea is not to dogpaddle around in a pool while hoping to get a date for Saturday night from a fellow club member, but to work out diligently. Check out the spa or health club before signing up. Make sure it has the kind of facilities that meet your needs. If the idea of soaking in a hot tub after the workout has enough appeal to motivate you to get to the gym, take that into consideration. Watch out for the hard sell. If a commission is involved, great pressure may be brought to bear on you to sign up on the spot. However, most health clubs have trial memberships and one day or week-long passes they will hand to you if you appear to be a serious prospect. Ascertain whether you are getting involved in a local, regional, or national (even international) facility. Most important, make sure, if you are joining a club for group support and professional guidance, that you will get it. Speak to the instructors and to other members.

The best approach, of course, is to participate in several physical activities throughout the week, with perhaps tennis one day, walking the next, and swimming the third. Whatever is convenient and reasonable. (You might want to check with your doctor before you begin, particularly if you are over forty years of age.) Different sports work different muscles. And while it is true that certain inherited traits and physical qualities (muscle fiber type, lung capacity, amount of body fat, heart size, and frame) can predispose you to do better at some activities than at others, anyone in good health can participate in *any* sport. Coordination will improve, appetite will lessen, your body will realign itself, and your muscles will firm up. The whole process should eventually become pleasurable. If it does not, then change activities. Try a different tactic. Have some fun during and after the actual diet process. While you are at it, your fat cells will become more mobile and begin migrating around your body rather than settling in problem "spots."[7]

Combine the exercise aspect with group support, even if that group consists of two—you and a friend—and you should be well on your way to never having to be obsessive about your weight again. Within a matter of days or weeks (depending upon how much weight you want to lose) you will find the entire focus of your dieting shifting from crazed calorie counting to casual monitoring of intake. You are going to be surprised at how easy dieting can be and at how much your life will change in the process. There is no reason to spend endless hours concerned about a pound or two or ten or twenty. The pounds will not come back. You *can* do it.

NOTES

1. F. Heinzelman and R. W. Bagley, "Responses to Physical Activity and Their Effects on Health Behavior," *Public Health Reports*, vol. 85:905–911, 1970.

2. Earl Ubell, "Health on Parade," *Parade Magazine*, 13 February 1983, p. 13.

3. Gail Perrin, "Good Diet, Exercise, Help as Person Ages," *The Oregonian*, 26 December, 1982, p. 8.

4. Beverly H. Butterworth, "Track Pioneer Makes Mark," *The Oregonian*, 10 March 1983, sect. 3M, p. 2.

5. Gay Gaer Luce, "Biological Rhythms in Psychiatry and Medicine," U.S. Department of Health, Education, and Welfare, Public Health Service, DHEW Publication No. (ADM)78–247, 1970, p. 57.

6. "Value of Exercise After a Meal Cited," *The New York Times*, Science Watch, 5 July 1983, Section C, p. 2.

7. Barbara Edelstein, M.D., as quoted in "The Waist-Away Bikini Diet—4 Weeks to a Wonderful Figure," *Harpers Bazaar*, May 1982, p. 123.

9

Pre-Diet Questions and Answers

In Anticipation of Beginning The 21st Century Diet

Although The 21st Century Diet itself is very straightforward and practical, the information leading up to the *design* of The 21st Century Diet is new and fairly intricate. The following answers to anticipated questions may prove helpful.

Q: May I substitute meals?

A: Occasionally. The key, however, is to limit those substitutions to "same day" specific meals and foods from the other two diet menus. Remember, you are "rotating" your foods in order to prevent food addiction and enhance food variety. Make sure you only exchange appropriate meals or days. And only occasionally. The 21st Century Diet is predicated on a predominance of calories during daylight hours when you need the energy most of all. Breakfast, in particular, is the time for refueling. Going from the 1600-Calorie Plan to the 800- or 1200-Calorie Plan shifts the caloric balance designed for your specific plan and may affect your basal metabolism needs.

Q: What if I am allergic to a food on The 21st Century Diet?

A: If you have been hospitalized for your reaction to this particular food, or if your symptom is so severe that it is life threatening, *do not* eat that food. However, bear in mind that bioecologists have found that rotating foods properly can virtually eliminate the symptoms of food allergies, and you may find that in time (as little as four days or as long as several months) your allergic reaction to a food has

104

disappeared. Also, although allergists do not know exactly why a person might be allergic to something as natural as a common food, they suspect that the problem may be tied to poor nutrition aggravated by the effects of environmental pollution. Tests have revealed that by building yourself up with vitamins and doing the best you can to lessen or avoid pollutants, you may allow your system to stabilize. Allergies could be eliminated. Read Chapter Twelve.

Q: May I eat out on The 21st Century Diet?

A: If you are invited to eat out, go ahead! Just limit yourself to the à la carte items or the entrees that correspond to the appropriate 21st Century meal. If you would have been eating filet of sole at home, order sole at the restaurant. Keep it simple and go light on the sauces. The 21st Century Diet is designed to be a little flexible. Just use common sense. You are not supposed to be tied to your home while on The 21st Century Diet.

Q: May I take diet pills?

A: Only for a day or two. Linda Wilcoxon Craighead, a psychologist, and her colleagues at Pennsylvania State University, organized a six-month study of the relative effectiveness for weight loss of diet pills and behavior modification. Some of the 120 women who participated were given the diet pill, while others learned techniques to change their eating habits. At the end of the six-month period the group taking the diet pills had lost the most weight. However, one year later they had regained 63 percent of the weight, whereas those participants on the behavior modification program alone regained only 17 percent of their lost weight. In other words, do not rely on diet pills to produce lasting results.

Theoretically, according to Dean Siegal, director of Thompson Medical Company, the chemical phenylpropanolamine (PPA) works because it acts on the hypothalamic area of the brain, not by curbing appetite per se, but by reducing sensitivity to taste and odor. Therefore, when the pills are no longer being taken, food regains its former taste, and old eating habits are resumed.[1] (As a note of interest PPA was originally developed as a nasal decongestant. Inadvertently, it was discovered to have an ability to suppress appetite.) After ten years of intensive research, PPA is now the most common ingredient in nonprescription diet pills. However, since pills reduce your interest in eating, you may not eat enough to maintain energy levels, and may therefore become lethargic. To counteract lethargy, caffeine is also added to many OTC (over the counter) diet pills. Because on The 21st Century Diet caffeine may be consumed only between the hours of 3 o'clock and 4:30 in the afternoon when it has a negligible effect, those diet pills cannot be taken! If you want to take a diet pill on the firt few days of The 21st Century Diet, feel free to do so, but *only* if it does not contain any caffeine. Diet pills may give you an extra boost to get started, and that is fine, but although the White House Special Action Office for Drug Abuse Prevention has not found that PPA has any potential for physiological habituation, no one is certain about the potential for "psychological" addiction. Why take the risk?

Q: I never eat breakfast and I cannot bear the thought of it. What should I do?

A: Eat it anyway. The 21st Century Diet is designed to be your lifetime diet. Since undoubtedly this is not your first diet, you are definitely doing something wrong. Begin doing something right by eating a high protein breakfast that will not only give you five hours of sustained energy, but will also eliminate your body's natural desire for a midmorning refueling. As Dr. Ernesto Pollit of the University of Texas School of Public Health in Houston reported, children who skipped breakfast were proved to have more difficulty in solving academic problems and made more errors (particularly in the late morning) than those youngsters who sat down to a breakfast before heading out for the school bus.[2] One in five people skips breakfast. Don't be one of them anymore.

Q: Exercise? Must I?

A: To exercise is an excellent idea. Although you will lose weight on The 21st Century Diet without exercising (and some people simply will not exercise), getting your body in motion has many benefits, not the least of which is to raise the basal metabolic rate and make weight loss easier. However, if you do not exercise, you *must* participate in a support program. Otherwise, you are just counting calories again. If a weight loss program is to be effective, it has been proved that you must do *more* than count calories. Although you must count calories, too. All over the world men and women are counting calories . . . and then recounting them a few weeks or months later. Limiting calories consumed during the day is essential, it will not be enough to produce lasting results. If you are not going to exercise, count your calories by selecting the appropriate plan *and* join a support group that is *fun*.

Q: I really hate to give up alcoholic beverages. I look forward to my cocktails before dinner and a glass or two of wine with dinner. Am I going to be able to drink on this program?

A: It is very important for men and women who drink alcoholic beverages to recognize that a form of food addiction that is also an allergy exists, and that alcoholic beverages contain food ingredients that are found every day in your diet. The ethyl alcohol in your favorite drink may not actually be what you want. The problem may be a desire to ingest certain food ingredients that are causing you mental or physical distress. It sounds complicated, but it is explained in detail in Chapter Seven. It is recommended that you not drink alcoholic beverages at all, but if you must, then limit yourself to *one* drink each day. A good fifteen to twenty percent of your daily caloric intake can be washed down in drink form, and can account for much of the extra weight you carry. Take a look at the amount of calories in alcoholic beverages. Then ask yourself how many alcohol-calories you normally consume each day. Think about it . . .

CALORIES IN ALCOHOLIC BEVERAGES

VARIETY	QUANTITY	CALORIES
Ale	8 ounces	150
Beer	8 ounces	120
Brandy	1 ounce	75
Champagne	6 ounces	175
Creme de Cacao	1 ounce	100
Creme de Menthe	1 ounce	100
Gin	1 ounce	75
Port	4 ounces	135
Sauterne	4 ounces	95
Scotch	1 ounce	85
Sherry	2.5 ounces	95

CALORIES IN ALCOHOLIC BEVERAGES *(cont'd.)*

VARIETY	QUANTITY	CALORIES
Sloe Gin	1 ounce	55
Vermouth	4 ounces	175
Vodka	1.5 ounces	180
Wine, dry	4 ounces	95
Wine, sweet	4 ounces	130

Also, very often when you first get home at night you are very dehydrated. Most people do not drink enough fluids throughout the day. At work or school, schedules simply do not permit the time or the opportunity. Yet, of the six classes of nutrients (protein, fat, carbohydrates, vitamins, minerals, water) water is the most important nutrient of all. You can survive for weeks without any of the other nutrients, but within a few days of going without water, you die. Take a look at the sketch below. Sixty percent of your weight is water. You must keep replenishing it.

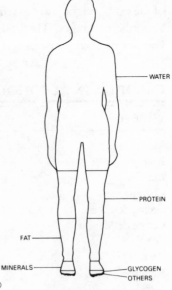

There is a good reason that diets call for large amounts of water consumption. Easily sixty percent of your body weight is water. Keep drinking it. It is quenching . . . and devoid of calories.

Source: From *Atlas of the Body and Mind.* Copyright © 1976 by Mitchell Beazley, Ltd. Published in the U.S. by Rand McNally and Company.

It is a good idea to drink a large glass of water when you first return home at night. Often, all those drinks after work could be reduced to one or two if your thirst was quenched prior to the first alcoholic beverage.

Q: When should I begin?

A: During a week when you will be doing little socializing. If that means putting the actual menus off for a while, do so. In the interim, proceed with the other aspects of The 21st Century Diet. As explained in Chapter Eight, as part of your approach to dieting you should join a support group and/or select physical activities that you might consider fun, and that will also encourage you to stay on the diet program. This is the way you are going to lose weight *and* keep it off.

Q: Are there any specific steps you might suggest just prior to beginning the diet?

A: Yes. Again, decide on the ancillary aspects of your diet. Will you be joining a group? Will you be getting into a sport or activity that you enjoy and that also encourages you to diet and reinforces your progress? Decide . . . and act. Then . . .

1. Dust off your scale and . . . step on! Jot down the bad news. By the way, digital scales are wonderful for watching yourself "flicker" between pounds as your weight level drops. Very encouraging! Plan to weigh in every day.

2. Check the foods in your kitchen cabinets against a list of the foods you will be needing for the first few days or first week of The 21st Century Diet. Buy as "close to natural" foods as possible. Get rid of those tempting foods. Don't eat them! Give them away or throw them away or freeze them! Remember, your family (if you do not live alone) should be participating in The 21st Century Diet, at least to the extent that they do not buy or insist that you buy their favorite and fattening foods, and that if they must, they should eat them off the premises! If worse comes to worst and you must have a few taboo items in the house, make them things you do not like.

3. When you do eat at home, if you live alone and are cooking for one, dish out one serving, and before you eat, quickly put any leftovers in the refrigerator. If you are cooking for more than one,

resist the buffet style serving. Give out individual servings that are sufficient for each person at the table. No more. No less. Dieting is a "family affair." If someone else is doing the cooking, reemphasize the information given in Chapter Five. Enlist everyone's cooperation.

4. When you do sit down to eat, relax, chew slowly, take small bites. Enjoy your food. In addition, scientists have discovered that a part of your brain called the hypothalamus plays a vital role in hunger pang control and sense of satiety. Until the hypothalamus receives a signal that food has entered your body (usually about twenty minutes from the first bite) you continue to feel "empty." Think about those occasions when you have eaten multicourse meals. After eating a few hors d'oeuvres, an appetizer, and a salad, the entree that sounded so appealing just three dishes back now isn't nearly so eagerly anticipated. Why? The digestive process has begun and enough time has elapsed from the first morsel so that the hypothalamus has received signals informing it that hunger should abate. It does, and you feel full. If you don't give the hypothalamus twenty minutes to register incoming nourishment, but instead eat as fast and furiously as possible, at the end of twenty minutes you'll have eaten much more food than you actually need.

5. It may sound old hat, but do drink lots of liquids. At the University of Maryland a study was performed that showed six to ten glasses of water or unsweetened tea (make it herbal) daily staved off hunger and helped people who normally confused thirst with hunger. Too often people have a quick drink at breakfast and lunch, then go all day without liquids.

6. Get into "constitutionals," those old-fashioned walks after meals. After lunch or supper get up and out. Take a walk around your office building or a stroll through the neighborhood. Get your blood circulating. Burn a few calories the easy way while you are at it. Too boring? Take a friend and chat along the way. Remember, these activities are supposed to be fun. You are supposed to be participating in enjoyable activities. Make them as frequent as possible for maximum benefits.

Now it is time to begin the actual 21st Century Diet plan. Get ready for an enlightening experience. By participating in a multiapproach method that takes the obsession out of counting calories and adds the fun ingredient of a support group and/or outside activities that assist weight loss, you are going to find The 21st Century Diet method surprisingly delightful.

If you fell into the category of a food addicted person, as explained in Chapter Seven, then you should have spent the last four days breaking that addiction on either the Food Elimination Method, the Rinkle Mono-Diet Method, or the Food Abstention Method. You, too, are ready for your "last" diet, The 21st Century Diet.

NOTES

1. Susan Duff, "Diet Pills Work?," *Mademoiselle,* July 1982, p. 46.
2. Jane E. Brody, "How Diet Can Affect Mood and Behavior," *The New York Times,* 17 November 1982, Section C, p. 16.

10

The 21st Century Diet
Plans and Menus

FACT: You should follow the 800 calories per day plan if you are short in stature and/or very sedentary.

FACT: You should follow the 1200 calories per day plan if you are of average height and/or moderately active.

FACT: You should follow the 1600 calories per day plan if you are extremely tall, exceptionally active and/or extraordinarily obese.

A Successful Diet = The Sum of Its Parts

The 21st Century Diet is unique in that it approaches weight loss from more than one angle. The 21st Century Diet keeps in mind not only the United States government's recommended daily allowances for ideal daily intake of protein, fat, and carbohydrates, but combines that information with the knowledge that vitamins, food rotation, and food variety, as well as support systems and, optionally, exercise, are crucial elements in a truly successful diet.

MEAL PLAN DESIGN

You will begin by cutting down on your previous daily intake of protein, and the protein you do eat will include a variety of sources besides meat, which is not only highly caloric, but also burdensome to your essentially omnivorous digestive tract. Also, your protein intake will occur mostly during the daylight hours when your energy needs are greatest. Since protein supplies you with the kind of sustained energy on which you need to draw to have a productive day, and decreases appetite better than carbohydrates, you will find The 21st Century Diet a relief from other diets that leave you watching the clock and anxiously biding your time until your next meal. Your predominantly high carbohydrate meals will be at night. Carbohydrates give you a quick boost of energy, and then allow you to sleep much more readily than does protein. Since carbohydrates are utilized more efficiently by your body in the evening, you can eat relatively large quantities of low calorie high carbohydrate foods . . . and fall blissfully asleep when the time comes.

You do not have to count the calories on the three plans, it is done for you. If you eat out, or if you simply want to eat more or less at a particular meal, you can switch to one of the other two plans randomly, as long as you switch a specific day and meal to the same day and meal on another plan. You will still lose weight, and not break your diet, although the rate at which you take weight off will depend on how often you substitute from another plan. The point is that you do not break or ruin the diet by upscaling to another meal from another plan, or by switching to another plan for an entire day. Just keep the specific days the same so you do not disrupt the rotation aspect of the diet by eating the same foods too frequently, and don't switch too often from your prescribed diet plan, which is based on your height, as well as your pre-diet weight and activity levels.

The 21st Century Diet Basic Rules

The following is an outline of the rules and regulations of The 21st Century Diet that apply equally to all three plans. As explained in Chapter Eight, now is the time to decide whether you will create or join a support group and/or continue or begin a calorie burning program of increased physical activity.

1. Eat all meals specified, including snacks. Your system is geared to foraging, and wants to nibble every hour and a half. By eating the occasional snacks when specified, you will satisfy what is essentially a prehistoric need.

2. Feel free occasionally to jockey back and forth between plans as long as you consistently switch to the same day on another plan. For example, Day #1 meals are for Day #1 only.

3. To avoid dehydration, drink a great deal of fluid, at least six or eight glasses each day.

4. Eat slowly. Scientists have located a hunger center called the hypothalamus in your brain. It takes twenty minutes from the time you take your first bite of food until the hypothalamus registers incoming food and makes you feel full.

5. Keep alcoholic beverages to a minimum, or better yet, do not drink them at all. Alcoholic beverages have little or no nutritional value, but lots of calories. If you are like the typical American adult for whom ten to twenty percent of daily calories is derived from alcohol, the alcoholic beverages you drink can be responsible for much of your excess weight. Also, alcohol is a classic releaser of inhibitions, working against most dieters' self-control. You know yourself. If you find you give into temptation more easily after a drink, don't drink.

6. Decaffeinated coffee or caffeine-free herbal teas are allowed anytime, as are caffeine-free, sugar-free diet sodas. Since caffeinated beverages have been proven to make you sleepy when you take them in the morning, and keep you awake at night, their consumption is restricted to the hours during which scientists have found that they do not cause any ill effects at all—between 3:00 and 4:30 in the afternoon.

7. You must take a multivitamin everyday. Wait until you have some food in your stomach, then take the vitamin with lots of water. See Chapter Twelve.

8. Try to select fresh foods that are as free from contaminants as possible, and as "close to natural" as they can be.

What to Expect

Initially, you can expect a dramatic drop in weight of several pounds—almost overnight—particularly, as explained in Chapter Seven, if periodic bloating (allergic edema) has been one of your problems. Dr. Donald Robertson of the South West Bariatric Clinic in Arizona attributes eighty percent of initial weight loss to fluid release. Expect those first few pounds, encouraging though they may be, to represent mostly water loss. A "true" pound of excess weight is only eliminated after you have consumed 4000 fewer calories than you have expended. You will be losing fractions of pounds unless your daily caloric intake was maintaining an enormous amount of extra weight. It may take a few days for your scale to reflect a drop in weight that includes fat as well as fluid.

After the first week you will invariably hit a plateau and linger at the same weight for a few days. Do not worry about it. The "pause" in your diet is only your body trying to enter a state of equilibrium to compensate for the rapid water loss the previous week. Do not get discouraged. Take it as a good sign that your system is stabilizing. Periodically thereafter, you may experience a day or two where you do not seem to lose any weight or the weight loss process slows down dramatically. There is some controversy over this situation. Some researchers theorize that you may be battling against your particular "set-point," or a balance between amounts of fat and muscle in your body, and at which weight your body would linger were you not dieting at all. Nevertheless, another day or two on The 21st Century Diet (preferably augmented with increased exercise), and you should break through all plateaus.

If you need to take a laxative every few days, feel free to do so. Your body will also be cleansing itself of toxins that accumulate when you diet. It is the build-up of these toxins that can make you feel weak and wobbly on a diet. Flush them out if your intestines are backed up. (The build-up of your body's natural waste products can also be responsible for what appears to be a weight plateau in your diet.) You will feel much better instantly.

Stop dieting when you reach the point where most of your weight is being carried in "lean" pounds or muscle. You should look trim and slim, and have renewed vigor and agility. Read Chapter Thirteen and find out how to maintain your ideal weight.

CHOOSING THE CORRECT 21ST CENTURY DIET PLAN

The following table is designed to help you choose just the right diet plan at the start of your weight reduction effort. Begin by checking the left-hand column for your height range, then assess your activity levels and overall weight problem. If at the start of The 21st Century Diet you are, say, of average height, but truly obese, then follow the 1600-calorie diet plan (as indicated) until you have lost sufficient weight to change categories. Once you are only about twenty pounds overweight, you may reassess your weight profile and your activity level, and switch to either the diet appropriate for the very athletic person, the moderately active person, or the sedentary person in your height category.

Indeed The 21 Century Diet is designed to be flexible enough to take into account an ever-changing schedule that permits or makes impossible physical activity that would normally burn off calories while, at the same time, you are counting (and reducing) them. Always, however, keep in mind your height, which determines minimums for basal metabolism needs.

If your height is	VERY ATHLETIC	MODERATELY ACTIVE	SEDENTARY	OBESE
Short	1600	1200	800	1600
Average	1600	1200	800	1600
Tall	1600	1600	1200	1600

The 1600-Calorie Plan
Extremely Tall, Exceptionally Active, and/or Extraordinarily Obese People

Sixteen hundred calories a day may sound like a great deal to a person who has participated in crash diets, high carbohydrate diets, high protein diets, liquid diets, etc., but in reality 1600 calories a day, while allowing rather elaborate and sumptuous meals, promotes substantial weight loss.

TALL DIETERS

The average woman stands about 5'5" tall and the average man approximately 5'8". If you are substantially taller than these figures, then there is no need to diet on less than 1600 calories a day unless you are extremely sedentary. You will lose plenty of weight . . . and quickly. Just maintaining enough weight to carry your height requires that you consume more calories than someone six inches shorter who weighs as much as you do.

ACTIVE DIETERS

Off season, an athlete expends far less energy than during practice sessions and actual games. He may weigh in at 250 pounds and be solid muscle at the end of the season, but unless he continues his level of activity or decreases his caloric intake, he is going to see muscle turn into fat and, since fat requires fewer calories to maintain, he is going to experience a weight gain. In a revealing three-week study showing how man's instincts control his body weight, psychologist Theresa Spiegle allowed participants to consume as much liquid diet drink (Metrecal) as they wanted throughout each day. The subjects had absolutely no idea how many calories were in each portion of liquid food they drank because they sipped the fluid through a tube that led to a hidden container. Within a few days most of the participants were consuming their normal number of calories each day, albeit in liquid form. After seven days Spiegle diluted the diet drink to one-half the calories. Again, most of the participants met their normal caloric intake—by drinking more.[1] Since a football player is used to consuming a certain number of calories a day to maintain his weight, if his activity level drops, he will have to adjust his caloric intake against his instincts. However, as long as his activity level does not drop to complete inactivity, 1600 calories per day will be sufficient to ensure significant weight loss and sufficient energy to facilitate exercise.

EXTRAORDINARILY OBESE DIETERS

In one of his best known works, *The Unquiet Grave,* published in 1945, Cyril Vernon Connolly (1903–1974) commented that "Inside every fat man a thin one is wildly signaling to be let out." Initially, weight gain starts out as simply eating more calories than you burn. Enormous weight gain does not happen overnight. It is the result of ever-escalating caloric intake and ever-decreasing physical activity.* In 99 out of 100 cases the truly "obese" are victims of the *addictive form of food allergy*,[2] and should turn to Chapter Seven before proceeding on any one of The 21st Century Diets. It is absolutely crucial to eliminate and break the grip of food addiction prior to commencing the diet plans. Answer the questionnaire. If you answer all the questions negatively then you may proceed with the 1600 calories per day plan. If you respond positively to one or more questions, however, take the four days necessary to break the chain of food addiction. It will be worth the effort, and enable The 21st Century Diet to be your last weight reduction diet.

---

*Think about swimming aerobics as a good exercise if you are extremely obese. You'll be buoyant in the water and able to do many exercises that would be impossible on land until you lost a great deal of weight. And in addition, you will activate your sluggish metabolism. Start somewhere . . . and swimming is potentially fun. Remember, fun is the important ingredient in successful dieting and weight maintenance.

1600 CALORIES PER DAY: MENUS*

DAY #1

Breakfast

eggs, chicken, 2 or quail, 10	cantaloupe, 1/2 or casaba melon, 1/2 or crenshaw melon, 1/2 or honeydew melon, 1/2 or Persian melon, 1/2	margarine, 2 Tbs.

Snack

	cashews, 16 or pistachio nuts, 60 or chestnuts, 6	

Lunch

tuna fish, 3 1/2 ounces (waterpacked) or flounder, 6 ounces	artichoke, 1 medium or lettuce tomato, 1 small	mayonnaise, 2 Tbs.

Snack

	apple, 2 or pear, 2	

Supper

crab, 2 1/2 ounces or shrimp, 3 ounces or rabbit, 2 ounces	yam, 1 medium or Chinese water chestnuts, 16 asparagus, 6 spears	margarine, 2 Tbs. honey, 1 Tbs.

*If you would rather have a food in its liquid form, see page 205 for some equivalents.

1600 CALORIES PER DAY: MENUS

DAY #2

Breakfast

puffed rice cereal,
    1 cup
and milk, 1 cup
    low-fat
or
Cheddar cheese,
    1½ ounces
or
muenster cheese,
    1½ ounces
or
Swiss cheese,
    1½ ounces

tangerines, 2
or
tangelos, 2

Snack

grapes, small bunch
or
papayas, 2

Lunch

turkey, 2 ounces
or
swordfish,
    3½ ounces
or
red snapper,
    3½ ounces

carrots, 3 large
or
parsnips, ¾ cup

margarine, 1½ Tbs.

Snack

bananas, 2 large
or
plantain, 1 5-inch
    fruit

1600 CALORIES PER DAY: MENUS

DAY #2

Supper

kasha/buckwheat, 1/2 cup (measured raw)	broccoli, 1 cup or cauliflower, 1 cup or Brussels sprouts, 8	margarine, 2 Tbs.
	walnuts, 8 mushrooms, 1 cup pineapple, 1 cup	

DAY #3

Breakfast

bacon, 4 slices or pork sausage, 2 links or scrapple, 3 1/2 ounces or ham, 3 1/2 ounces	sesame crackers, 8 or macadamia nuts, 6

Snack

	blueberries, 1 cup or cranberries, 1 cup or guavas, 2

Lunch

salmon, 4 ounces or rainbow trout, 4 ounces or haddock, 5 ounces or mackerel, 5 ounces	avocado, 1/2 or brazil nuts, 8 or squash, 2 cups or watermelon, 1 half-inch slice	margarine, 2 Tbs.

1600 CALORIES PER DAY: MENUS

DAY #3
Snack

peaches, 2
or
plums, 2
or
raspberries, 1 cup
or
strawberries, 1 cup
or
apricots, 4
or
cherries, 30 large

Supper

lobster, 3 1/2 ounces	potatoes, 2 large	margarine, 2 Tbs.
or	or	
sole, 3 1/2 ounces	eggplant, 1 1/2 cups	
or	or	
venison, 2 1/2 ounces	green peppers, 3	

DAY #4
Breakfast

oatmeal, 1 cup	grapefruit, 1
cooked	or
or	oranges, 2
herring, 3 1/2 counces	or
or	kumquats, 8
sardines, 3 1/2 ounces	
or	
goose eggs, 2	

Snack

figs, 2
or
mulberries, 1 1/2 cups
or
prickly pears, 2

1600 CALORIES PER DAY: MENUS

DAY #4

Lunch

rib lamb chop, 1 lean	spinach, 1 1/2 cups	margarine, 2 Tbs.
or	or	
bluefish, 3 1/2 ounces	beets, 1 cup	
or		
abalone, 3 1/2 ounces		
or		
halibut, 3 1/2 ounces		

Snack

	pomegranate, 1 cup
	or
	elderberries, 1 cup
	or
	gooseberries, 2 cups
	or
	olives, 8 green

Supper

clams, 2 large	sweet potato, 1 cup	margarine, 2 Tbs.
or	or	
mussels, 2 ounces	okra, 36 pods	
or		
scallops, 1 1/2 ounces	coconut, 1/2 cup, fresh	
or	or	
tofu (soya curd), 3 1/2 ounces	dates, 7	

The 1200-Calorie Plan
Average Height and/or Moderately Active People

When determining which 21st Century Diet plan to employ, take height and activity level into account as separate entities. The 1200-Calorie Plan is ideal for those men and women who are of average height *and/or* who will be moderately active while on The 21st Century Diet. If you are a short, sedentary person who does not plan to maintain or increase his or her physical activity, then the 800-Calorie Plan is the one for you. If you are really tremendously overweight, there is no need to cut back to 800 calories or to 1200 calories per day at this stage. The 1600-Calorie Plan will produce extraordinary results, but without such a drastic caloric reduction.

Remember, physical activity burns calories and, although as explained in Chapter Five, gender, age, and previous history of dieting are factors influencing the number of calories required daily to maintain your weight levels, 1200 calories constitutes a significant reduction in overall calories compared to the amount you must consume every day in order to maintain your present weight. (A 154-pound woman sustains that weight on about 2300 calories per day. A man sustains 220 pounds on about 3700 calories per day.) However, if you are physically active, whether that means pumping iron at the local gymnasium or walking twenty minutes to work and twenty minutes back each day, and you can maintain or increase your level of physical activity while on the 1200-Calorie Plan, the effect will be as if you were actually consuming far fewer than 1200 calories per day. *Burning* calories while at the same time *reducing* caloric intake not only denies your system incoming and fat producing food, but simultaneously stimulates your metabolism to burn already stored fat.

Also, feel free to switch *occasionally* to meals on the 800-Calorie Plan if your schedule precludes exercise that day. If you are eating out or having guests over and want to prepare a somewhat more lavish meal, feel free to substitute a meal from the 1600-Calorie Plan. You will continue to lose weight. After all, a female who wants to weigh 121 pounds will eventually maintain that weight by eating 1650 to 1950 calories per day, depending upon her activity levels and age! A 165-pound male can sustain his weight by eating foods containing from 2500 to 2950 calories per day! A 1600-calorie day or one of the specific meals from that plan is not going to ruin the diet. Remember, however, that The 21st Century Diet has a food rotation aspect to it, so you must be very careful to substitute meals from the same day—Day #1 lunch on the 800-Calorie Plan for Day #1 lunch on the 1200-Calorie Plan, for example.

1200 CALORIES PER DAY: MENUS*

DAY #1
Breakfast

eggs, chicken, 2 or quail, 10	cantaloupe, 1/2 or casaba melon, 1/2 or crenshaw melon, 1/2 or honeydew melon, 1/2 or Persian melon, 1/2	margarine, 1 Tbs.

Snack

	cashews, 6 or pistachio nuts, 30 or chestnuts, 3

Lunch

tuna fish, 3 1/2 ounces (waterpacked) or flounder, 6 ounces	artichoke, 1 or lettuce, unlimited tomato, 1 small	mayonnaise, 2 Tbs.

*If you would rather have a food in its liquid form, see page 205 for some equivalents.

1200 CALORIES PER DAY: MENUS

DAY #1
Snack

apples, 2
or
pears, 2

Supper

crab, 2½ ounces	yam, 1 medium	margarine, 1 Tbs.
or	or	
shrimp, 3 ounces	Chinese water	
or	chestnuts, 16	
rabbit, 2 ounces		
	asparagus, 6 spears	

DAY #2
Breakfast

puffed rice cereal,	tangerines, 2
1 cup	or
and milk, 1 cup	tangelos, 2
low-fat	
or	
Cheddar cheese,	
1½ ounces	
or	
muenster cheese,	
1½ ounces	
or	
Swiss cheese,	
1½ ounces	

Snack

grapes, small bunch
or
papayas, 2

1200 CALORIES PER DAY: MENUS

DAY #2
Lunch

turkey, 2 ounces	carrots, 2 large	margarine, 2 tsp.
or	or	
swordfish,	parsnips, ½ cup	
3½ ounces		
or		
red snapper,		
3½ ounces		

Snack

	bananas, 2 large
	or
	plantain, 1 5-inch
	fruit

Supper

kasha/buckwheat,	broccoli, ½ cup	margarine, 2 tsp.
¼ cup	or	
(measured raw)	cauliflower, ½ cup	
	or	
	Brussels sprouts, 4	
	walnuts, 4	
	mushrooms, ½ cup	
	pineapple, ½ cup	

DAY #3
Breakfast

bacon, 4 slices
or
pork sausage, 2 links
or
scrapple, 3½ ounces
or
ham, 3½ ounces

1200 CALORIES PER DAY: MENUS

DAY #3

Snack

blueberries, 1 cup
or
cranberries, 1 cup
or
guavas, 2

Lunch

salmon, 3½ ounces	avocado, ¼	margarine, 2 Tbs.
or	or	
rainbow trout, 3½ ounces	Brazil nuts, 4	
or	or	
haddock, 4½ ounces	squash, 2 cups	
or	or	
mackerel, 3½ ounces	watermelon, 1 quarter-inch slice	

Snack

peaches, 2
or
plums, 1
or
raspberries, ½ cup
or
strawberries, ½ cup
or
apricots, 3
or
cherries, 15 large

Supper

lobster, 3½ ounces	potato, 1 large	margarine, 2 Tbs.
or	or	
sole, 3½ ounces	eggplant, 1½ cups	
or	or	
venison, 2½ ounces	green peppers, 3	

1200 CALORIES PER DAY: MENUS

DAY #4

Breakfast

oatmeal, 1 cup cooked or herring, 3 1/2 ounces or sardines, 3 1/2 ounces or goose eggs, 2	grapefruit, 1/2 or orange, 1 or kumquats, 4

Snack

	figs, 2 or mulberries, 1 1/2 cups or prickly pears, 2

Lunch

rib lamb chop, 1 lean or bluefish, 3 1/2 ounces or abalone, 3 1/2 ounces or halibut, 3 1/2 ounces	spinach, 1 1/2 cups or beets, 1 cup	margarine, 1 Tbs.

Snack

	pomegranate, 1/2 cup or elderberries, 1/2 cup or gooseberries, 1 cup or olives, 4 green

1200 CALORIES PER DAY: MENUS

DAY #4
Supper

clams, 2 large	sweet potato, ½ cup	margarine, 1½ Tbs.
or	or	
mussels, 2 ounces	okra, 18 pods	
or		
scallops, 1½ ounces	coconut, ½ cup, fresh	
or	or	
tofu (soya curd), 3½ ounces	dates, 7	

The 800-Calorie Plan
People Short in Stature and/or Very Sedentary

The 800-Calorie Plan is an approach to taking pounds off that produces dramatic results without jeopardizing your health. Everyday you will consume approximately 800 calories, but no less. It is important not to skip meals or snacks, or attempt an even more rapid weight loss by cutting meals on this plan. George F. Cahill, M.D., of the Harvard Medical School, has discovered a protein-sparing mechanism that comes into play automatically when your body goes without *any* incoming food. As if a switch were thrown, after a day or two of not eating, your body draws on its own reserves and nonvital supplies, and at the same time suppresses your appetite and hunger pangs. Depending upon the size of your reserves, you can live for weeks without food before entering a state where lack of food could cause death, though you must have water every day. However, if you do continue to eat, but consume fewer than 800 calories per day, it is biochemically impossible for your protein-sparing switch to be thrown, and you rapidly enter a state of physical starvation that can be very serious. In addition, by eating a little, but not enough, you are constantly ravenous.

There is a significant difference between being *undernourished* and being *malnourished*. In the case of undernourishment, you can cut calories and, if you have a nutritionally sound diet, remain essentially healthy. Whereas, you can also eat many thousands of vitamin-, mineral-, and protein-deficient calories each day, and be malnourished. Malnutrition is not caused by lack of food, but rather by inferior quality and improper balance of food. Undernourishment involves a lack of calories that exists when caloric intake falls far below the body's energy needs for an extended period. Of course, both conditions can exist simultaneously. For example, people in countries where food is scarce can suffer from acute vitamin, mineral, and protein deficiency as well as food deprivation. (Children with distended abdomens display a classic sign of protein deficiency or malnourishment and, if the children are also emaciated, they are undernourished as well.) When cutting calories drastically, you do not want to become malnourished at all or undernourished in the extreme. In the case of severe undernourishment your body would begin to draw on its own muscle and internal organs for nourishment. However, as long as your metabolic needs are met sufficiently by *minimum caloric intake* that is accompanied by sufficient proportions of protein, fat, and carbohydrates, as well as the proper amount of essential vitamins, minerals, and trace elements, you remain perhaps underfed, but still well fed. And, as you enter the process of weight loss, your body will quite naturally turn to its own fat reserves to maintain your energy levels. *The key figure is 800 calories per day.* By allowing yourself at least 800 calories per day, researchers have found you will not "shock" your system into a starvation response.

Of course, if you are overweight by tens of pounds or hundreds of pounds, or very athletic, you will see results that are nearly as dramatic by scaling up to the 1600-Calorie Plan. Ideally, the 800-Calorie Plan should be employed by those adults who are battling a maximum weight problem of twenty-five pounds, not a two hundred pound weight load. For the dieter with a severe weight problem there is no need for such a severe cutback in caloric intake to get fine results, and if you have been constantly dieting and redieting over the years, a steady, higher calorie plan may be better suited for stabilizing your metabolic rate.

800 CALORIES PER DAY: MENUS*

DAY #1
Breakfast

eggs
  chicken, 2
  or
  quail, 10
	cantaloupe, 1/4
	or
	casaba melon, 1/4
	or
	crenshaw melon, 1/4
	or
	honeydew melon, 1/4
	or
	Persian melon, 1/4	

Snack

	cashews, 6 or pistachio nuts, 30 or chestnuts, 3	

Lunch

tuna fish, 3 1/2 ounces (waterpacked) or flounder, 5 ounces	artichoke, 1 medium or lettuce, unlimited tomato, 1 small	mayonnaise, 1 Tbs.

Snack

	apple, 1 or pear, 1	

Supper

crab, 2 1/2 ounces or shrimp, 3 ounces or rabbit, 2 ounces	yam, 1 medium or Chinese water chestnuts, 16 asparagus, 6 spears	margarine, 1 tsp.

*If you would rather have a food in its liquid form, see page 205 for some equivalents.

800 CALORIES PER DAY: MENUS

DAY #2

Breakfast

puffed rice cereal, 1 cup and milk, 1 cup low-fat or Cheddar cheese, 1½ ounces or muenster cheese, 1½ ounces or Swiss cheese, 1½ ounces	tangerine, 1 or tangelo, 1

Snack

	grapes, small bunch or papayas, 2

Lunch

turkey, 2 ounces or swordfish, 3½ ounces or red snapper, 3½ ounces	carrots, 2 large or parsnips, ½ cup	margarine, 1 tsp.

Snack

	banana, 1 large or plantain, half a 5-inch fruit

800 CALORIES PER DAY: MENUS

DAY #2
Supper

broccoli, 1/2 cup or cauliflower, 1/2 cup or Brussels sprouts, 4 walnuts, 4 mushrooms, 1/2 cup pineapple, 1/2 cup	margarine, 2 tsp.

DAY #3
Breakfast

bacon, 4 slices
or
pork sausage, 2 links
or
scrapple, 31/2 ounces
or
ham, 31/2 ounces

Snack

blueberries, 1/2 cup or cranberries, 1/2 cup or guava, 1

Lunch

salmon, 31/2 ounces or rainbow trout, 31/2 ounces or haddock, 41/2 ounces or mackerel, 31/2 ounces	avocado, 1/4 or Brazil nuts, 4 or squash, 2 cups	margarine, 1 tsp.

800 CALORIES PER DAY: MENUS

DAY #3
Snack

peaches, 2
or
plum, 1
or
raspberries, 1/2 cup
or
strawberries, 1/2 cup
or
apricots, 3
or
cherries, 1/2 cup

Supper

lobster, 31/2 ounces	potato, 1 large	margarine, 1 tsp.
or	or	
sole, 31/2 ounces	eggplant, 11/2 cups	
or	or	
venison, 21/2 ounces	green peppers, 3	

DAY #4
Breakfast

oatmeal, 1 cup cooked	grapefruit, 1/2 medium
or	or
herring, 31/2 ounces	orange, 1
or	or
sardines, 31/2 ounces	kumquats, 4
or	
goose eggs, 2	

Snack

fig, 1
or
mulberries, 3/4 cup
or
prickly pear, 1

800 CALORIES PER DAY: MENUS

DAY #4
Lunch

rib lamb chop, 1 lean	spinach, 1½ cups	margarine, 2 tsp.
or	or	
bluefish, 3½ ounces	beets, ½ cup	
or		
abalone, 3½ ounces		
or		
halibut, 3½ ounces		

Snack

	pomegranate, ½ cup
	or
	elderberries, ½ cup
	or
	gooseberries, 1 cup
	or
	olives, 4 green

Supper

clams, 2 large	sweet potato, ½ cup	margarine, 1 Tbs.
or	or	
mussels, 2 ounces	okra, 18 pods	
or		
scallops, 1½ ounces		
or		
tofu (soya curd),		
3½ ounces		

Substitute Foods*

The following foods have *not* been used in organizing the 21st Century Diet menus; therefore, they may be used as substitute foods on any day for any meal—as long as the protein content and caloric content approximate the food you are replacing. (See the Appendix for protein and caloric content of *all* foods.) Remember, however, not to eat any of the substitute foods more frequently than once every four days or any food from the same family of foods more frequently than every other day.

SUBSTITUTE FOODS
Approximately 3½ Ounces or a Little Less than ½ Cup

ANIMALS	Calories	Protein (grams)	Carbohydrates (grams)
Anchovy Family			
anchovies, 12 thin	84	9.6	trace
Barracuda Family			
barracuda	113	21.0	0.0
Catfish Family			
catfish	103	17.6	0.0
yellow bull head	103	17.6	0.0
Croaker Family			
croaker	96	17.8	0.0
drum, red	80	18.0	0.0
sea trout	195	21.5	0.0
silver perch	—	—	—
spot	219	17.6	0.0
weakfish	121	16.5	0.0
Diamondback Terrapin Family			
diamondback terrapin	—	—	—
green turtle	89	19.8	0.0
Dove Family			
dove	—	—	—
pigeon (squab)	142	17.5	0.0

*Note: The only omissions from this list are those entire food families for which no caloric, protein, and carbohydrate information is available at this time.

SUBSTITUTE FOODS
Approximately 3½ Ounces or a Little Less than ½ Cup

ANIMALS	Calories	Protein (grams)	Carbohydrates (grams)
Eel Family			
eel	233	15.9	0.0
Frog Family			
bull frog (4 legs)	73	16.4	0.0
Guinea Fowl Family			
guinea fowl	158	23.4	0.0
eggs	—	—	—
Harvestfish Family			
butterfish	169	18.1	0.0
harvestfish	95	16.2	0.0
Herring Family			
roe, shad	130	42.4	1.5
Jack Family			
amberjack	—	—	—
jack mackerel	143	21.6	0.0
pompano	166	18.8	0.0
yellow jack	—	—	—
Minnow Family			
carp	115	18.0	0.0
chub	145	15.3	0.0
Muskellunge Family			
northern pike	—	—	—
pickerel	84	18.7	0.0
Octopus Family			
octopus	73	15.3	0.0
Opossum Family			
opossum	221	30.2	0.0
Oyster Family			
oyster, 8	66	8.4	3.4
Perch Family			
perch, yellow	91	19.5	0.0
pike	84	18.7	0.0
sauger	84	17.9	0.0
walleye	93	19.3	0.0
Porgy Family			
scup (porgy)	112	19.0	0.0

SUBSTITUTE FOODS
Approximately 3½ Ounces or a Little Less than ½ Cup

ANIMALS	Calories	Protein (grams)	Carbohydrates (grams)
Scorpionfish Family			
rosefish (ocean perch)	88	18.0	0.0
Sea Bass Family			
bass, yellow	88	18.0	0.0
grouper	87	19.3	0.0
perch, white	91	19.3	0.0
sea bass	96	21.4	0.0
Silverside Family			
mullet	146	19.6	0.0
silverside	—	—	—
whitebait	—	—	—
Smelt Family			
smelt	98	18.6	0.0
Squid Family			
squid	84	16.4	1.5
Sturgeon Family			
beluga	—	—	—
sturgeon caviar	262	26.9	3.3
Sucker Family			
bigmouth buffalofish	113	17.5	0.0
black buffalofish	113	17.5	0.0
sucker	104	20.6	0.0
Sunfish Family			
black bass species	93	19.2	0.0
bluegill	—	—	—
sunfish species	—	—	—
longear sunfish	—	—	—
pumpkinseed	—	—	—
crappie	79	14.6	1.2
Tilefish Family			
tilefish	79	17.5	0.0
Whale Family			
whale	156	20.6	0.0
Whitefish Family			
lake whitefish	155	18.9	0.0

SUBSTITUTE FOODS
Approximately 3 1/2 Ounces or a Little Less than 1/2 Cup

PLANTS	Calories	Protein	Carbohydrates
Birch Family			
filbert (hazelnut),			
10-12 nuts	97	1.6	3.0
Carpetweed Family			
New Zealand spinach	19	2.2	3.1

NOTES

1. Flora Davis, "News," *Mademoiselle,* July 1982, p. 54.
2. Marshall Mandell, M.D., and Lynne Waller Scanlon, *Dr. Mandell's 5-Day Allergy Relief System* (New York: T. Y. Crowell, 1979), p. 116.

11

Mid-Diet Questions and Answers

Just prior to the beginning of The 21st Century Diet and occasionally during the diet, it is a good idea to read and reread the Question and Answers chapters. Inevitably, periodic questions will arise, especially as you become more and more involved in the weight reduction process. The following questions and answers should provide the information you are seeking after starting your diet.

Q: I have lost fifteen pounds on the 1200-Calorie Plan in three weeks. My face and shoulder areas are starting to look very gaunt, and friends and co-workers are beginning to tell me to stop the diet, that I have lost enough. But my goal is another ten pounds. Should I quit? I really am looking pinched.

A: Do not quit yet. If your goal is to drop ten more pounds, go to it. During the rapid weight loss process, it is not unusual for the face and shoulder area to get very thin, very quickly. However, within just a few weeks—four at the most—after you end the weight reduction aspect of your diet, your remaining fat will redistribute . . . and your face and shoulders will fill in a bit. Far too many people quit dieting too early because of the surprise of looking in the mirror and seeing what looks like a sunken face. Keep dieting. Everything will balance out later.

Q: I am so overweight that it is depressing, and I know you want me to exercise, but I cannot seem to find any enthusiasm for anything because of my weight. How can I get started?

A: No one but you can drag yourself out of your lethargy. What it will take is a commitment at least to give an activity the chance to prove itself. Some dieters find that if they make the commitment to a weekend bicycle trip, or create a vacation agenda that includes physical activities such as hiking or tennis or soccer, the act of preparing the plan provides the momentum necessary to carry it out and then continue the activities afterward. You have to use some imagination. Check the Optional Athletic Activities list in Chapter Eight. Pick a few activities and try them out. Also, bear in mind that exercise stimulates the pituitary gland in the brain, which in turn produces high levels of beta endorphin, which in turn acts as a natural antidepressant and mood elevator. That's why people get, in a sense, addicted to exercise and their daily workout. Give it a try.

Q: What if I fall off The 21st Century Diet?

A: Get back on right away and don't worry about it. Actually, for some unknown reason women seem to be much harder on themselves than men when it comes to breaking a diet. When a woman indulges in a food that is taboo on a diet, often she topples off her diet for days, even weeks or months at a time. To her, breaking the diet is a major catastrophe. Men, however, seem to have a much more matter-of-fact attitude toward a forbidden slice of pizza. One meal "off" and the next meal "on." To men, a slip off a diet is simply a minor setback. A lapse should not mean a relapse.

Q: My spouse and I exercise together on The 21st Century Diet, but I seem to be losing weight faster than she. How come?

A: There are physiological reasons for your losing more weight. Size counts: A 275-pound person walking two miles per hour burns 6.4 calories per minute. A 150-pound person walking at the same speed only burns 3.5 calories per minute. Gender counts, too: if you and your wife are the same height, you, the male, would burn more calories faster simply because of your ratio of muscle to fat. Men have a higher ratio of muscle to fat, and muscle requires more calories to maintain. In addition, the female hormones, estrogen and progesterone, are "fat hoarding" and "fat producing" substances.

Q: I am convinced that exercise will make me even hungrier than I usually am. It seems that about one hour after jogging, I am ravenous. Am I right?

A: According to Howard F. Hunt, chairman of the physical education department at the University of California at San Diego, exercise does not increase appetite, but it "increases your sense of taste. . . ." Other authorities feel that there is an initial increase in appetite after starting an exercise program, but that the net effect of routine exercise is reduced food intake.[1]

Q: Should I take a laxative?

A: Some dieters experience constipation while on a new eating regimen. If your problem is constipation, do not suffer with it. Feel free to take a mild laxative every few days for the first week or two, and no longer. Chronic use of laxatives causes constipation. You do not want to get caught in that situation. Within a week or two your system should have stabilized. Also, drink lots of fluids throughout the day. Too many people, dieting or not, barely drink any fluids until the evening hours.

Q: I notice you allow diet pills for the first few days on The 21st Century Diet. How about starch blockers?

A: Forget it. Starch blockers are supposed to inhibit the digestive enzyme amylase, which in turn stops the body from processing starch. Claims have not been substantiated by any legitimate scientific research to date. What is known, however, is that starch blockers are made from the extract of beans. Beans cause flatulence, cramps, and even diarrhea in many people. To boot, undigested starch, lingering in the digestive system, provides a banquet for bacteria normally found in the intestines. These bacteria also produce flatulence as a by-product.

Q: How much salt should I put on my food?

A: Evolutionary evidence suggests that the need for salt is not only biological, but instinctive, and may be directly related to mankind evolving from the sea (a very salty place!). Dr. Derek Denton, director of the Howard Florey Institute of Experimental Physiological and Medicine in Melbourne, Australia, has performed research with salt-deprived sheep. After a few days without salt, the sheep drank salt water—but just enough to restore their proper salt levels, not enough to make them ill. Because they drank the salt water so quickly and then just as quickly ceased drinking, Dr. Denton felt that the signal the sheep got to stop drinking was instinctive, since the salt did not even have the time to reach the sheep's tissues before the animals' "thirst" was quenched.[2] Like the human preference for sweet-tasting and high protein foods, the craving for salt may be one that is indulged excessively because of easy access to salt shakers and salty foods.

You do need salt (sodium chloride) to maintain your proper blood volume, to control the flow of water in and out of your body cells, to assist in the transmission of nerve impulses, to help metabolize food, to control the body's acid balance, and to aid in the action of certain enzymes. During a leisurely day without much physical activity, the National Academy of Science indicates that you need a minimum of approximately 1100 milligrams (or about ½ teaspoon) of sodium chloride daily. If you are extremely active, 3000 milligrams (or about 1½ teaspoons) is desirable. The average person in the United States gets 6,100 to 18,000 milligrams each day! That's five teaspoons or 10 grams each day, 3 of which are from the natural salt content of food, 4 from processed food, and 3 from cooking and adding salt at the table. Use salt sparingly. Your taste buds really will adjust. Also, watch out for foods like frankfurters (627 mg or ⅓ teaspoon in one 2-ounce portion), corned beef (1,474 mg or ⅔ teaspoon in 4 ounces), soy sauce (1,379 mg or ⅔ teaspoon in 1 tablespoon), pickles (928 mg or ½ teaspoon in 1 medium dill), and frozen vegetables. Frozen vegetables, in particular, have been found to contain 100 percent more salt than fresh vegetables.[3]

Q: Must I prepare meals exactly as specified?

A: No. However, keep in mind the ingredients and measurements of what is scheduled that day if you are going to innovate. Also, should you want to avoid a particular ingredient if, for example, you are allergic to it, feel free to do so, but bear in mind that you want to maintain high protein breakfasts and lunches and predominantly high carbohydrate suppers. Remember, too, that you are rotating your foods so you will not be eating any two foods from the same family of foods that day, such as a banana and a plantain (both Banana Family foods). Pick the substitution from the variety of different food families offered that day, but choose items that do not appear on the specific menu plan.

Q: I don't always feel that I have the time to eat the required snacks on The 21st Century Diet. Is it all right to skip them occasionally?

A: No. The 21st Century Diet is based on your daily body rhythms, and they call for a bit of nibbling about every one and one-half hours. In addition, a piece of fruit or a handful of nuts is nourishing, adds a boost of energy, and help stave off any hunger pangs that might tempt you to stray from the actual diet plan. Moreover, you may be surprised at just how satisfying a simple snack can be.

Q: I developed a migraine headache on Wednesday right after I ate lunch. Did the diet cause my migraine?

A: Not the diet per se, but a food on the diet may be the culprit. Bioecologists have found that foods, chemicals, dusts, animal danders, and beverages you come across every day can be the cause of migraine headaches. What bioecologists have also discovered is that when you avoid the food to which you are allergic for a number of days, your migraine clears, but you then become even more sensitive to the food that was causing the migraine in the first place. The acute sensitivity begins after four days of not encountering the food, and lasts in varying degrees from weeks to months thereafter. (Reread Chapter Seven for more information about allergies.) What probably happened is that through the food rotation process you stopped eating a "problem" food and entered a stage of acute sensitivity. The good news is that you can be pretty confident that you now know at least one of the causes of your migraine—a food you ate at lunchtime. Now you have a choice: eat the food again the next time it rotates by on the menu and see what happens, or substitute a food. If you opt for the former and get a migraine, you will confirm the allergy, and if you decide to substitute a food and do not get a migraine, you will also have good evidence that one or more of those lunchtime foods may have caused the migraine. Ideally, you should take this information to an allergist who can test you sublingually (under the tongue) with an extract from the foods you suspect. Refer to the List of Bioecologists in the United States in Chapter Seven. Write them and find out if there is a physician in your area whom they can recommend.

Q: May I improvise recipes?

A: Absolutely. For example, when The 21st Century Diet calls for a combination of vegetables, plus a dab of margarine, feel free to sauté your vegetables, or steam them and add the margarine. You are being given the ingredients but it is up to you to concoct the meal you desire. Use whatever spices you like as well. They do not contain any calories. Add any you want. For example, if you want to have curried chicken, that's fine. Or broiled chicken with paprika. Use your imagination.

Q: Not all the foods (ham, for example) are allowed by my religion. What should I do on the days that call for pork?

A: Do the same thing that a person who is allergic to a food has to do: select one of the other foods offered as an option or choose a food that does not appear on the menu that day already, but is allowed on the list of substitutions. Keep your substitution within the same range of protein or carbohydrate content as the food you are replacing. Use the Food Families list in the Appendix to help you determine portion, etc.

Q: Sometimes the menus call for a specific amount of food, for example $3\frac{1}{2}$ ounces. Must I measure?

A: First-time dieters (and most men!) seem blissfully unaware of caloric content—until they start measuring. Often it comes as a great shock to them to discover that certain foods are significantly higher in calories than other foods, and that size of serving can make or break a diet. Measure initially, just to see the quantity involved in $3\frac{1}{2}$ ounces . . . or one cup. Get yourself an inexpensive food scale, or adapt a scale used for weighing letters.

Q: Fish for breakfast?

A: The 21st Century Diet is designed to supply you with the majority of your calories and the major portion of your protein intake earlier in the day, when you most need the energy that calories and protein supply. Unlike Europeans and Asians, who do not find it unusual to eat fish and other high protein foods at breakfast, too many Americans typically are light breakfast eaters . . . and predominantly high carbohydrate breakfast eaters. The exception may be the American farmers who would not think of eating a sugar doughnut or one slice of bread for fuel for a morning's work in the fields. Those types of breakfasts are akin to putting jet fuel in a Volkswagen; you skyrocket for a few minutes, then blow your engine.

Everybody should eat a hearty breakfast to ensure lots of physical energy as well as maximum mental acuity. As explained in detail earlier, scientific testing has proved this to be the case. Sweet breakfasts or predominantly high carbohydrate meals simply don't make the grade.

Q: What do I do about determining caloric content of brand-name foods?

A: Purchase a calorie guide that specializes in brand-name foods. Any bookstore will have one.

Q: Opossum? Bison? Snake? Quail? Turtle? Deer? Where am I supposed to get these oddball foods?

A: What to you sounds far-fetched may be the usual fare for someone in another part of the country. For example, men and women who live in rural areas may find they have access to foods that are far different from the foods found in suburban communities. Interestingly, urbanites often have a tremendous selection from which to choose—if they make the effort to do a little research. (Big, ethnically mixed cities will have grocery stores that cater to the tastes of the various communities.) Buffalo no longer roam solely in the West or in zoos. Hugh and Joan Forbes have a small herd of them in New Castle, Pennsylvania, and serve buffalo burgers at their drive-in restaurant. The National Buffalo Association says that buffalo burgers, steaks, and roasts are twenty-five percent higher in protein than beef cattle, and are cholesterol-free.[4] And it is tasty; in a restaurant in New York City called An American Place one of the hors d'oeuvres that was much in demand was buffalo sausage, sliced, dipped in crumbs, and fried.[5] Horsemeat is another high-protein food possibility that has found favor among Europeans and Asians. Although horse lovers in the United States tend to take to the streets with picket signs when they get wind that supermarkets are carrying horse steak, in reality horse steak is high in protein, priced well below beef, and delicious to boot. So while it may seem shocking at first to you to think that turtle is a choice on The 21st Century Diet, for some dieters it will be simply a case of digging down to the bottom of the freezer!

Your best bet when trying to locate foods not found commonly in your supermarket or at the local butcher store is to open up the yellow pages of the phone directory and look under "Food." There will be subheadings such as "Game, fresh and frozen" or "Gourmet." Just a glance will tell you whether you will be able to obtain certain foods locally from suppliers in your area or whether you will have to order by mail. Bear in mind that if you do have to place an order that must be shipped to you that there will be shipping costs. If the food you order is frozen, such as quail or pheasant or fish from faraway places, it will have to be sent via some sort of overnight carrier service. Therefore, it is recommended that you buy in larger quantities and have a big enough freezer to accommodate the shipment. Another approach might be for you and friends or neighbors to get together and divide the costs and share storage space. In neighborhoods that have butcher stores or friendly supermarket managers, you might be able to arrange to have them make the actual purchase if enough people show interest.

Here's a list of a few mail-order companies specializing in the more exotic or difficult-to-obtain foods. All these companies ask of you is a little time to get the more elusive items (lion meat!), to bear in mind that some items are more seasonal than others, and that you should order in sufficient quantities to make it worth everyone's while, including yours:

American Spoon Foods 411 East Lake Street Petoskey, Michigan 49770 (616) 347-9030	buffalo meat sausage, muskrat, game birds, dried morel mushrooms . . . almost anything given notice.
Schumann de Mer Corp 18 Monterey Drive Manhasset Hills, New York 11040 (212) 821-2600	conger eel, frog legs, lake barracuda, kippers (herring), caviar, duck, rabbit, venison, quail eggs, rattlesnake meat

Chevalean Foods
PO Box 803
666 Winsor Street
Hartford, Connecticut 06101
(203) 246-8518

USDA Grade A "table quality" horsemeat in steaks and patties

Flying Foods International
158-08 Rockaway Blvd.
Jamaica, NY 11434
(212) 706-0820

wild Texas boar, axis venison, Scotland hare, duck, partridge, fruits and vegetables

Iron Gate Products Co., Inc.
424 West 54th Street
New York, New York 10019
(212) 757-2670

rabbit, duck, lion, pheasant, quail, reindeer, venison, all varieties of fish

Beck Sausage, Inc.
South Park Route
Box 2141
Jackson, WY 83001
(307) 733-8343

buffalo meat

Manchester Farms
P.O. Box 97
Dalzell, SC 29040
(803) 469-2588

quail and eggs

Signature Prime
143 South Water Market
Chicago, IL 60608
(800) 621-0397

pheasants, squab, partridges, brown bear, antelope, venison, wild goat, and llama

---

The following is a list of people and markets that specialize in the more ethnically oriented foods. If you are interested in Chinese, German and Austrian, Indian and Ceylonese, Indonesian, Japanese, Middle Eastern, Scandinavian, South American, Mexican and Caribbean foods, contact retailers who specialize in food from these faraway places.

MISCELLANEOUS

Martin's Gift Basket Shop, 1264 Third Avenue, New York, NY
10021   (212) 288-7716

Maryland Market, 412 Amsterdam Avenue, New York, NY
10024   (212) 595-1224

William Poll's Gourmet Shop, 1051 Lexington Avenue, New York,
NY 10021   (212) 288-0501

Crescent Market, 6409 Avondale, Oklahoma City, OK 73116
                                                           (405) 842-2000

John Wanamaker, 1300 Market Street, Philadelphia, PA
19139   (215) 422-2000

J. Goldsmith Department Store, 123 S. Main Street, Memphis, TN
38103   (901) 529-4545

Simon David, 7117 Inwood Road, Dallas, TX 75209
                                                           (214) 352-1781

CHINESE

Kwong On Lung Company, 680 N. Spring Street, Los Angeles,
CA 90012   (213) 628-1069

Wing Chong Lung Company, 922 S. San Pedro Street, Los
Angeles, CA 90015   (213) 627-5935

Manley Produce, 1101 Grant Avenue, San Francisco, CA
94133   (415) 928-1490

Shing Chong and Company, 800 Grant Avenue, San Francisco, CA
94108   (415) 982-0949

Shiroma, 1134 W. Argyle Street, Chicago, IL 60640
                                                           (312) 561-5794

Star Market, 3349 N. Clark Street, Chicago, IL 60657
                                                           (312) 472-0599

Wing Fung Lin, 79 Harrison Avenue, Boston, MA 02111
                                                           (617) 542-2449

Eastern Trading Company, 1123 Broadway, New York, NY
10010   (212) 924-2308

Wing Fat Produce Company, 193 East Broadway, New York, NY
10002   (212) 964-1030

Oriental Import-Export Company, 2009 Polk Street, Houston, TX
77003   (713) 223-5621

GERMAN AND AUSTRIAN
Bremen House, 218 East 86th Street, New York, NY 10028
(212) 288-5500
Karl Ehmer Quality Meats, 230 East 86th Street, New York, NY
10028   (212) 535-2129
Schaller and Weber, 1654 Second Avenue, New York, NY
10028   (212) 879-3047

GREEK
Daldas, 199 Eddy Street, San Francisco, CA 94102
(415) 775-5065
Maletis Brothers, 100 Northwest Third Avenue, Portland, OR
97209   (503) 227-0718

HUNGARIAN
Jossef Mertle, 1508 Second Avenue, New York, NY 10021
(212) 744-8292
Paprikas-Weiss, 1546 Second Avenue, New York, NY 10028
(212) 288-6117
H. Roth and Son, 1577 First Avenue, New York, NY 10028
(212) 734-1110

INDIAN AND CEYLONESE
Bezjian Grocery, 4725 Santa Monica Boulevard, Los Angeles, CA
90029   (213) 663-1503
Haig's, 441 Clement Street, San Francisco, CA 94118
(415) 752-6283
Central Grocery Company, 923 Decatur Street, New Orleans,
LA 70116   (504) 523-1620
Progress Grocery Company, 915 Decatur Street, New Orleans, LA
70116   (504) 525-6627
Delmar Foods, 501 Monroe Avenue, Detroit, MI 48226
(313) 961-5504
Kalustyan Orient Export Trading Corp, 123 Lexington Avenue,
New York, NY 10016   (212) 685-3416
Antone's, 2606 Sheridan, Tulsa, OK 74129   (918) 835-5519
Jamail's, 3114 Kirby Drive, Houston, TX 77006   (713) 523-5535

House of Rice, 4112 University Way NE, Seattle, WA 98105
(206) 633-5181

INDONESIAN
Holland American Market, 10343 East Artesia Boulevard,
Bellflower, CA 90706   (213) 867-7589
Yee Sing Chong, 966 North Hill, Los Angeles, CA 90012
(213) 626-9619
Haig's, 441 Clement Street, San Francisco, CA 94118
(415) 752-6283
Wing Sing Chong, 1076 Stockton Street, San Francisco, CA
94108   (415) 982-4171
Granada Fish Market, 2400 Broadway, Denver, CO 80202
(303) 249-0126
Tuck Cheong, 802 Seventh Street NW, Washington, DC
19801   (202) 842-1114
Holland Dutch, 6917 West Roosevelt Road, Berwyn, IL
60402   (312) 484-6899
Cardullo's Gourmet Shop, 6 Brattle Street, Cambridge, MA
02138   (617) 491-8888
Wah Lee Company, 3409 Cass Avenue, Detroit, MI 48201
(313) 831-8660
House of Rice, 4112 University Way NE, Seattle, WA 98105
(206) 633-5181

ITALIAN
Manganaro Brothers, 488 Ninth Avenue, New York, NY
10018   (212) 563-5331
Paul Urbani, 130 Graff Avenue, Trenton, NJ 08638
(609) 394-5851

JAPANESE
Modern Food Market, 318 E. Second Street, Los Angeles, CA
90012   (213) 488-0611
Pacific Mercantile Company, 1925 Lawrence Street, Denver, CO
80202   (303) 295-0293

Diamond Trading Company, 913 W. Belmont, Chicago, IL
60657   (312) 472-5520
Franklin Food Store, 1309 East 53rd Street, Chicago, IL
60650   (312) 493-5057
Oriental Merchandizing Company, 2636 Edenborn Avenue,
Metairie, LA 70002   (504) 888-3191
Yoshinoya, 36 Prospect Street, Cambridge, MA 02139
                                                     (617) 491-8221
Oriental Trading Company, 10525 J Street, Omaha, NE
68510   (402) 331-5511
Katagiri Company, 224 East 59th Street, New York, NY
10022   (212) 755-3566
Tanaka and Company, 326 Amsterdam Avenue, New York, NY
10023   (212) 874-6600
Soya Food Products, 2356 Wyoming Avenue, Cincinnati, OH
45214   (513) 661-2250
Omura Japanese Food and Gift Shop, 3811 Payne Avenue,
Chicago, IL 44114   (216) 881-0523
Anzen Importers, 736 Northeast Union Avenue, Portland, OR
97232   (503) 233-5111
Sage Farm Market, 1515 S. Main Street, Salt Lake City, UT
84101   (801) 484-4122
Uwajimaya, Inc., 422 South Main Street, Seattle, WA 98104
                                                     (206) 624-6248

MIDDLE EASTERN
Europa Grocery Company, 321 South Spring, Los Angeles, CA
90013   (213) 628-4873
Haig's, 441 Clement Street, San Francisco, CA 94118
                                                     (415) 752-6283
Greek American Grocery Company, 2690 SW 22nd Street,
Miami, FL 33129   (305) 854-7468
Central Grocery Company, 923 Decatur Street, New Orleans, LA
70116   (504) 523-1620
Progress Grocery Company, 915 Decatur Street, New Orleans, LA
70116   (504) 525-6627

Cardullo's Gourmet Shop, 6 Brattle Street, Cambridge, MA
02138   (617) 491-8888
George Malko, 182 Atlantic Avenue, Brooklyn, NY 11201
                                                        (212) 642-2049
Sahadi Importing Company, 187 Atlantic Avenue, Brooklyn, NY
11201   (212) 624-4550
House of Yemen East, 370 Third Avenue, New York, NY
10016   (212) 532-3430
Kalustyan Orient Export Trading Company, 123 Lexington
Avenue, New York, NY 10016   (212) 685-3416
Stamoolis Brothers Grocery, 2020 Penn Avenue, Pittsburgh, PA
15222   (412) 471-7676
Barzizza Brothers, 315-353 South Front Street, Memphis, TN
38103   (901) 332-8390
Merlino Fine Foods, 2822 Rainier Avenue South, Seattle, WA
98144   (206) 723-4700

SCANDINAVIAN
Nyborg and Nelson, 153 East 53rd Street, New York, NY
10022   (212) 223-0700
Old Denmark, 133 East 65th Street, New York, NY 10021
                                                        (212) 744-2533

SOUTH AMERICAN, MEXICAN, AND CARIBBEAN
Jurgenson's Grocery, 133 Larchmont Boulevard, Los Angeles, CA
90004   (213) 469-1901
Casa Lucas Market, 2934 24th Street, San Francisco, CA
94110   (415) 826-4334
Mi Rancho Market, 3365 20th Street, San Francisco, CA
94110   (415) 647-0580
Pena's Spanish Store, 1636 17th Street NW, Washington, DC
20009   unlisted
Epicure Markets, 1656 Alton Road, Miami Beach, FL 33139
                                                        (305) 672-1861
La Preferida, 177-181 West South Water Market, Chicago, IL
60608   (312) 666-5858

Marshall Field and Company, 111 North State Street, Chicago, IL
  60602   (312) 781-3668
Swiss Colony, Lindale Plaza, Cedar Rapids, IA 52402
                                                         (319) 393-9132
Central Grocery Company, 923 Decatur Street, New Orleans,
  LA 70116   (504) 523-1620
Progress Grocery Company, 915 Decatur Street, New Orleans, LA
  70116   (504) 525-6627
Cardullo's Gourmet Shop, 6 Brattle Street, Cambridge, MA
  02138   (617) 491-8888
Continental Gourmet Shop, 210 S Woodward Avenue,
  Birmingham, MI 48011   (313) 642-5236
Casa Moneo Spanish Imports, 210 West 14th Street, New York,
  NY 10011   (212) 432-2720
Spanish American Food Market, 70001 Wade Park Avenue,
  Cleveland, OH 44103   (216) 432-2720
Morris Zager, 221 Sixth Avenue North, Nashville, TN 37207
                                                         (615) 255-3108
Jamail's, 3114 Kirby Drive, Houston, TX 77006
                                                         (713) 523-5535
Pier 1 Imports, 5403 South Rice Avenue, Houston, TX
  77036   (713) 666-4387

Of course, the above is by no means an exhaustive list. Every state
will have a variety of stores that cater to the tastes of its populace.
The more diverse a state's or a county's mix of cultures, the more
variety in plant and animal foods will be on the shelves.

NOTES

1. A. S. Leon, J. Conrad, D. B. Hunninghake, R. Serfass, "Effects of a Vigorous
Walking Program on Body Composition, and Carbohydrate and Lipid Metabolism of
Obese Young Men," *American Journal of Clinical Nutrition*, 32:1776-87, 1979.

2. Harold M. Schmeck, "Hunger for Salt Found to Be Powerful Instinct," *The New
York Times*, 9 August 1983, Section C, p. 7.

3. Kathleen Stein, "Dr. C.'s Vitamin Elixers," *Omni*, April 1982, p. 70.

4. Staff reporter, "Buffalo Roaming Outside the West," *The New York Times*, 10
August 1983, Section A, p. 19.

5. Florence Fabricant, "Food Notes," *The New York Times*, 7 December 1983,
Section C, p. 4.

12

To Supplement or Not to Supplement

FACT: Your doctor may say you do not need vitamin and mineral supplements, but your doctor is *wrong*.

FACT: Your food has been depleted of as much as sixty percent of its natural vitamin content by the time it reaches your table.

FACT: You should buy *synthetic* supplements rather than *natural*.

FACT: You will be amazed at the amount of increased energy you have after just a week or two of taking a daily supplement.

The Dwindling Controversy

Up until a few years ago physicians all around the world were involved in a heated debate about the pros and cons of vitamin and mineral supplements to the diet. The vast majority of doctors felt that the vitamins and minerals found "naturally" in the foods people were eating every day were sufficient to keep mind and body healthy, and that there was no cause for alarm, let alone supplements. As time passed, however, evidence grew indicating that physical and mental problems were indeed being caused by the lack of adequate amounts of vitamins and minerals in the diet. Increasing numbers of doctors as well as specialists in allied fields, such as nutrition, began to reassess their stand. Now, more and more patients find that their physicians are recommending a daily supplement . . . and more and more people are finding their entire health picture improving from the moment they take their first multivitamin.

157

Even men and women who think they are healthy because they cannot pinpoint any specific problem related to a lack of vitamin and mineral supplements find that within a short time multivitamins make them feel more vigorous. Their nagging but not pressing minor ailments, such as slight eczema, acne, dry skin, chronic fatigue, reduced attention span, and the like can clear almost miraculously after a regimen that includes supplements. Within three months—the minimum amount of time if takes for your body to replace "old" cells with "new" cells in a cell turnover process—the results of adding essential vitamins and minerals to the diet become obvious, not only to the person who has an improved sense of well-being, but often to family members and friends who can notice the renewed vitality.

The first vitamin to be identified, vitamin A, was discovered in 1911 by a Polish biochemist, Casimir Funk. Since then, forty-eight various substances are recognized as requisite for optimal health. Without all the necessary vitamins and minerals, health and performance become impaired, affecting glands, nerves, blood vessels, and your digestive system—in short, your entire body. At first the problems are subtle, akin to running on only "four cylinders" of a six cylinder engine; you're still functioning, but not at optimal levels. Gradually, the symptoms of deficiency make their presence felt, but only after enough time has passed for enzyme function to be so dramatically affected that clinical indications are present.[1]

Vitamins! Vitamins! Vitamins!

In a college lecture series, nutritionist Paavo Airola, Ph.D., stressed that there was the "therapeutic versus the preventive approach" to diet. The former concerns curing and correcting the negative effects of a poor diet and the latter is designed to build, maintain, and sustain optimal health.[2] Although there is little starvation in America, malnutrition is rampant. In two studies of people who routinely ate a "good mixed diet," based on U.S. Recommended daily allowances, the Department of Agriculture found sixty percent malnourished.[3]

Poor nourishment opens the lid on a Pandora's box of potential health problems. In a revealing study that took place fifty years ago, Weston A. Price, D.D.S., partner in the Price-Pottinger Nutrition Foundation, investigated the effects of the "civilized diet" on fourteen primitive societies still scattered around the globe. As a dentist, he was particularly interested in before and after effects of a change in diet on teeth. Upon initial examination of tribespeople prior to the introduction of the modern diet, he was very impressed by their cavity-free and perfectly aligned teeth. Very rare, indeed, were dental-related problems. In addition, Price described the people he examined as appearing to be in a state of mental and physical health that was superior to that of western society. As time passed, and more and more of the primitive tribes came into contact with the civilized societies, the members of the tribes began to eat less and less fresh, unprocessed, locally available foodstuffs and switched more and more to refined and processed foods that are typical of American fare. Granulated sugars, bleached white flour, polished rice, canned fruits, and refined vegetable oils all became part of their diet. To Price, on his next examination, the most obvious indication that their health was being adversely affected by their modern diet was the *immediate* appearance of dental decay and susceptibility to infection in adult members of the tribe. In addition, for the first time in the history of the tribe, newborns had deformities that included club feet, cleft palates, crowded teeth, and narrowed dental arches.[4] Since the major problem with "civilized diets" is that the food is vitamin- and mineral-depleted, the participants in the study were reintroduced to their old, natural diet in an effort to reverse the damage done by inferior quality food. The result was that subsequent children of mothers who had given birth to malformed offspring were fine. They, unlike their brothers and sisters, had excellent teeth and normal facial structure. Poor maternal nutrition, thanks to the modern diet, had affected the earlier children with lifelong problems.

Of course, the reassuring aspect of this study is that, if caught in time, malnourishment in the first generation of adults experiencing it can be reversed in midstream. However, if you realize that you, your parents, and your grandparents are probably just links in an entire familial chain of malnutrition, the extent of the problem becomes more pronounced. Simple yet brilliant studies by Dr. Price's partner, Francis Pottinger, M.D., confirm the seriousness of the problem, while simultaneously offering hope. Pottinger examined cats over a four-generation period. Since cats are true carnivores, they require raw food in order to maintain maximum health and, as it turned out in Pottinger's studies, reproduce normally. Hypothesizing that a change in the "natural" diet of the cats might produce interesting results, Dr. Pottinger altered the 100 percent raw food diet to two-thirds cooked and one-third raw for the first generation of cats he studied. Immediately, the health picture of the cats began to alter and, ultimately, their longevity was reduced. Continuing the experiment to the grandchildren of the first cats studied, Dr. Pottinger found that within six months of birth, significant problems became evident. The females were far less fertile and had many more miscarriages than normal. In addition, they had allergies (an increase from five percent in the first generation to ninety-five percent), arthritis, lethargy, skin eruptions, decaying teeth, diabetes, pneumonia, nephritis, infections, intestinal parasites, as well as noticeable changes in attitude that included marked viciousness and homosexuality.[5] As in Price's experiments, Pottinger returned the third generation of experimental cats to their natural raw diet to see if he could reverse the inherent health problems of the cats. The bad news is that it took *three to four more generations* of eating proper foods to undo the damage wrought by a diet of unnatural foods. The good news was that the problems could be corrected at all.

Some people with severe mental problems have been helped most dramatically by megavitamin therapy, and have been rescued from lifelong residence in institutions as well as endless hours on the psychiatrist's couch. The disease called pellagra was found to be the result of a vitamin deficiency. The discovery that vitamin B-3 (niacin) deficiency was at the root of the disease that first caused dermatitis, then diarrhea, followed by dementia (psychotic behavior), and ultimately death, was a shock and a revelation to the medical community. Unfortunately, most traditional physicians refuse—or forget—to make the logical inference about vitamin B-3 deficiency: that somewhere before the onset of severe symptoms of the disease there is a very gray area in which the person's health profile begins to change in subtle and not yet observable ways. The patient is not yet "clinical," and yet not "well" either. After the onset of the dermatitis and through the final stages of dementia and death, many patients are misdiagnosed as incurable, when they should be receiving therapeutic doses of vitamin B-3.[6]

Beriberi is a vitamin deficiency disease which, at advanced stages, produces an enlarged heart, heart failure, and neuritis (inflammation of the nerves). A dramatic cure for beriberi is thiamine or vitamin B-1. Knowing that these symptoms can be a sign of B-1 vitamin deficiency, there is no doubt that patients in "heart failure" or suffering from painful neuritis could theoretically benefit from immediate therapeutic doses of vitamin B-1, which is a nontoxic and essential vitamin.[7]

The reason most physicians used to give for discouraging the use of vitamin and mineral supplements was their presumption that the foods produced and readily available to man are vitamin rich. Recent investigations show that this presumption is unfounded.

From Garden to Gullet

One of the most pressing problems faced by mankind today is the quality of the food commonly available. Produce may look healthy and appealing, meat may appear to be of a high quality, but both have severe inadequacies that can aggravate man's vitamin and mineral deficiencies.

The problem has its origins in the soil that produces the plants that are not only eaten by man, but also used as feed for animals that man will eat. Centuries ago, farmers knew nothing about vitamins and minerals, but they did realize that in order to produce robust crops, fields had to be rotated periodically. A field that lay fallow for a season or two seemed to produce a higher quality of plant the following season. It would take a while for scientists (and farmers) to realize that the plants were drawing "something" out of the soil in order to grow. That something was vitamins, minerals, and trace elements. When the chemical industry created products to destroy the pests and weeds that made crop failures a nightmare for farmers, they literally sterilized the soil by destroying the tiny microscopic bacteria and organisms that contribute natural vitamins, minerals, and trace elements to the soil. To recreate the balance of nutrients that the soil originally provided and the plants needed, the chemical industry developed synthetic or manmade fertilizers (vitamins and minerals). Research ultimately produced chemicals that enabled farmers to produce more crops, bigger crops, and healthier looking crops, but a problem existed because no matter how diligently the chemists tried to duplicate mother nature, they missed the mark. Foods are now "vitamin enriched," but not vitamin complete. And foods are certainly not embellished sufficiently to compensate for the estimated two to three percent vitamin depletion that occurs at every stage of the many processes and procedures between harvesting and your dinner plate. All told, fifty to sixty percent of the inherent vitamins and minerals can become dissipated.[8]

Dr. Michael Colgan of the University of Auckland, a visiting professor at Rockefeller University, attempted to assess the vitamin and mineral content of foods eaten every day in the American diet and purported to contain common levels of vitamins and minerals. Dr. Colgan was surprised to discover that the orange, supposedly rich in vitamin C, could vary from containing "only traces of vitamin C" to up to 180 mg of vitamin C per orange.[9] Such variations make it extremely difficult to determine the amount of supplements you should take. "RDAs," the United States government's recommended daily allowances, do not take into account the differing levels of inherent vitamins and minerals from one orange to the next. More-over, they are based on the premise that you are completely healthy to begin with. Stress, growth, gender, size, activity levels, infection, colds, allergies, alcohol consumption, drug intake, oral contraceptives, aging, artificial additives, food coloring, cigarette smoking, and environmental pollution all add to the basic nutritional needs of man, but RDAs do not take them into account. In bioassays (sophisticated tests that analyze the nutritional status of blood) of people who were considered "healthy," more than one-half of the participants were found to be deficient in vitamin E and one-third were lacking in one or more of the B vitamins (in particular, folic acid). Several of the people involved in the survey showed only "marginal levels" of B-12 and vitamin A. Fully half of the people showed signs of calcium and magnesium deficiency, and half the women were obviously lacking in "sufficient dietary iron." Almost one-third were too low in iodine. What is most shocking is that these apparently healthy individuals were already taking vitamins![10] As Senator William Proxmire described RDAs in 1977, "At best the RDAs are only a recommended allowance at antediluvian levels designed to prevent some terrible disease. At worst they are based on conflicts of interest and self-serving views of certain portions of the food industries. Almost never are they provided at levels to provide for optimum health and nutrition."

The Ideal Nutritional Supplement

Scurvy, the disease that was capable of killing sailors who put to sea for any length of time, was found to be selective in its victims. An entire crew could suffer lack of vitamin C for months at a time, and yet not everyone would develop scurvy. Those unfortunate mariners who succumbed were obviously people whose bodies required more vitamin C than those who lived. In other words, nutritional supplements should be custom tailored to take into account a person's specific dietary needs, which can vary quite considerably from individual to individual.

Although your bionutritional individuality can be determined through blood, urine, hair, and tissue analyses, these tests will only establish whether you are functioning at suboptimal levels—a condition already recognized as being generally true for the entire populace.[11] In addition, biochemical analysis will not reveal what your optimal levels should be. In fact, although determining maximum nutritional supplements for livestock is now a science in itself, no conclusive research data is available on optimal nutritional levels for individuals or even for man as a species.

The best you can hope to do right now, until researchers are able to say with relative certainty that they know the answers, is to ingest supplements made of a formula that contains the proper vitamin, mineral, and trace elements. In addition, try to eat foods that are considered as "close to natural" as possible (and therefore grown in naturally richer soil and not subjected to all the various vitamin-depleting processes that are part of "agribusiness" procedures) in order to stack the odds in your favor in case there should exist more nutrients yet to be discovered by scientists. After all, vitamin B1 was discovered before vitamin B2, vitamin B3, etc; and science is always evolving.

Synthetic vs. "Natural" vs. Artificial Supplements

The planet earth itself, and all its plants and animals, including man, are composed of naturally occurring chemicals. Water, for example, is a natural chemical that often contains varying amounts of dissolved vitamins and minerals as additional chemicals. The human body and all its organs are made from water, protein, fat, minerals, glycogen, and a variety of other "chemicals," such as nucleic acids. In general, chemicals can be divided into four categories: those that are naturally occurring (in plants, animals, and minerals); those that are formulated entirely from manmade sources (but which exactly duplicate the molecular structure of naturally occurring chemicals); those that are also formulated entirely from manmade sources (but are "artificial" in that they are not the molecular duplicates of any naturally occurring chemical on earth); and those that are made from the combination of naturally occurring and manmade sources (that could be combinations of exact molecular duplicates or artificial chemicals). "Synthetic" chemicals are either exact molecular duplicates of a naturally occurring chemical or the creation of new and artificial chemicals; both are produced by man in a laboratory.

When it comes to vitamin supplements, however, you have two choices: the naturally occurring vitamin that is ostensibly extracted entirely from various natural sources, or the synthetically derived vitamin that is indistinquishable in molecular composition from the naturally occurring vitamin. Which should you choose? The answer lies in the definition of "natural," as used by vitamin manufacturers and as allowed by the government, and in the cost differential. The following is a list of problems associated with "natural" vitamins.

Natural does not mean 100 percent. Even though a label may entice you into buying the product because of its natural qualities, beware. Very often the product contains far fewer natural ingredients than you might suspect. For example, vitamin C described as being from "rose hips" can actually consist of a perponderance of vitamin C *synthesized* originally from sugar. Since fresh rose hips contain only two to three percent vitamin C, to fulfill your minimum daily requirements you would need to eat fistfuls of tablets consisting entirely of processed rose hips powder. At the present time there is no federal regulation governing the use of the word "natural," either in terms of labeling or with regard to advertising. Food and drug regulations only specify that some percentage of a vitamin labeled as "natural" contain that vitamin in unsynthesized form. Therefore, drug companies are free to perpetrate this ruse on you.

Synthetic vitamins duplicate natural vitamins AND cost less. When pantothenic acid was discovered and isolated in the laboratory, one teaspoonful was secured from $20,000 worth of human effort and hundreds of pounds of beef liver. To obtain even one milligram each day of naturally occurring pantothenic acid, you would have to spend at least $2000. Synthesized pantothenic acid, however, duplicates exactly, through the wizardry of science, the original natural product at a tiny fraction of the cost. This naturally occurring form and the synthetic version are so precisely similar that, according to its discoverer, Dr. Roger J. Williams, former president of the American Chemical Society, and director of the Clayton Foundation Biochemical Institute at the University of Texas (where more vitamins and their variants have been discovered than in any other laboratory in the world), they can't be told apart by biochemists [the experts]. Since natural vitamins are already largely synthetic, it would be wise to head straight for the synthetic vitamins in the first place. Labeled as such, they are always less expensive. In the case of rose hips, so-called natural vitamins can be as much as two-and-a-half times more expensive.

Natural does not mean uncontaminated. When vitamins are produced synthetically in a laboratory, they emerge in tablet or capsule form free from various toxic chemical agents such as pesticides, herbicides, and insecticides that permeate natural food sources. Organic soil does not, by the way, guarantee that plants will be uncontaminated. Soil quality may be improved, but to eliminate all chemical residue is virtually impossible. In addition, weather conditions and time of harvest can have a positive or negative effect on the inherent quality of the final product. Synthetic vitamins, as compared to natural, are pure in every sense of the word. They have never touched soil and never been exposed to agricultural runoff of chemicals.

Starting or Switching Vitamins

Any vitamin is better than no vitamin. Even though optimal levels are not known yet, some research has been done to indicate minimal levels; however, these figures do vary according to source, and often from country to country.[12] Dr. Roger J. Williams developed what he calls the Vitamin and Mineral Insurance Formula. The formula is intended to supplement your diet in order to meet at least minimum daily requirements. Bronson Pharmaceuticals has decided to produce the formula, and has made it available by direct mail, thus avoiding the middleman and the resultant price markup. Their address is 4526 Rinetti Lane, La Canada, California 91011.

The Vitamin and Mineral Formula is based on that described in *The Physicians' Handbook of Nutritional Science* and in *The Wonderful World Within You*, written by Dr. Williams. As a note of interest, Dr. Williams does not derive any personal financial benefit from Bronson Pharmaceuticals. Dr. Williams published his formula simply to advise the medical community that he had developed one. It was Bronson Pharmaceutical's idea to produce it.

You can purchase the Vitamin and Mineral Insurance Formula in quantities of 100 and 250, at a price substantially below that of vitamins sold over the counter in drug stores, health stores, and grocery stores. Unlike most vitamin supplements, the tablets are free of flavoring, starch, artificial coloring, and sugar. As a result, the Vitamin and Mineral Insurance Formula is ideal for people with allergies. If you cannot swallow pills, there is no problem. Bronson has duplicated Dr. Williams's formula in chewable form, ideal for children as well as adults. One of the other advantages of the Vitamin and Mineral Insurance Formula is that the daily dosage is divided into three tablets. Since at first some people cannot tolerate a full dosage at once without developing heartburn and nausea, among other symptoms, you can start with one tablet and build your

VITAMIN AND MINERAL INSURANCE FORMULA

	ONE TABLET CONTAINS:	THREE TABLETS PROVIDE:
A (Palmitate)	2,500 IU	7,500 IU
D (Cholecalciferol)	133.4 IU	400 IU
E Alpha Tocopherol (as DL-Alpha Tocopheryl Acetate)	13.4 IU	40 IU
C (Ascorbic Acid)	83.4 mg	250 mg
B-1 (Thiamine Mononitrate)	0.67 mg	2 mg
B-2 (Riboflavin)	0.67 mg	2 mg
B-6 (Pyridoxine Hydrochloride)	1 mg	3 mg
B-12 (Cobalamin Concentrate)	3 mcg	9 mcg
Niacinamide	6.67 mg	20 mg
Pantothenic Acid (D-Calcium Pantothenate)	5 mg	15 mg
Biotin	0.1 mg	0.3 mg
Folic Acid	0.134 mg	0.4 mg
Choline (Bitartrate)	83.4 mg	250 mg
Inositol	83.4 mg	250 mg
Para-Amino-Benzoic Acid	10 mg	30 mg
Rutin	83.4 mg	250 mg
Calcium (Calcium Phosphate)	83.4 mg	250 mg
Phosphorus (Calcium Phosphate)	83.4 mg	250 mg
Magnesium (Magnesium Oxide)	66.7 mg	200 mg
Iron (Ferrous Fumarate)	5 mg	15 mg
Zinc (Zinc Gluconate)	5 mg	15 mg
Copper (Copper Gluconate)	0.67 mg	2 mg
Iodine (Kelp)	0.05 mg	0.15 mg
Manganese (Manganese Gluconate)	1.67 mg	5 mg
Molybdenum (Sodium Molybdate)	0.034 mg	0.1 mg
Chromium (Chromic Sulfate)	0.34 mg	1 mg
Selenium (Selenium Dioxide)	0.0067 mg	.02 mg

SUGGESTED DOSAGE:

Adults and Teen-agers: Three tablets daily.
Children 6–12 years: Two tablets daily.
Children under 6 years: One tablet daily (confirm with pediatrician).

tolerance levels slowly. Do not take them on an empty stomach. Wait until about twenty minutes after you have eaten. Then you have the option of taking all three at once, or staggering them throughout the day. A little trial and error will help you decide which plan you prefer.

A multivitamin instead of a handful of tablets from varying sources assures you that you are getting the proper balance of vitamins and minerals. Although each vitamin performs a specific task that cannot be duplicated by another vitamin, vitamins work synergistically, as a team, and therefore must be in balance. The absence of even *one* vitamin can cause biochemical disruption. Some vitamins do not get absorbed into your body unless accompanied by other vitamins. It can get very complicated. Your best bet is to let those men and women who have devoted their professional lives to the intricacies involved make the decisions for you.

Again, any vitamin supplement (synthetic) is likely to improve your overall health, but when dieting, it is especially important to supplement your foods. Many dieters have found that weakness due to rapid weight loss can be eliminated completely by taking a daily multivitamin. In a study performed by Dr. M. Colgan, ten out of thirteen patients on a diet reported that symptoms of weakness, tremor, and dizziness that they always associated with dieting disappeared when they took vitamin and mineral supplements.

Small Amounts Can Make Big Differences

Even people who feel they are in good health need vitamin and mineral supplements. No one, no matter how careful he or she is about his or her diet, can get away with not taking supplements and expect to be in optimal health. Not in today's world; not since United States government studies revealed that sixty percent of the people who ate what was considered a good "mixed diet" based on Recommended Daily Allowances (RDAs) showed clinical symptoms of malnutrition—regardless of their income levels.[14]

Even though you may not believe you have symptoms associated with lack of adequate vitamins and minerals, you do. It is called "subclinical walking malnutrition" and "selective starvation." Even a minute difference in dosage can make a profound difference in your mood and sense of well-being. In a recent study reported by the San Francisco conference of the American Fertility Society, twelve out of fourteen women who were unable to conceive a child for periods from one and one-half years to seven years became pregnant within months of taking prescribed amounts of vitamin B-6 each day.[15] In another study four experienced marathon racers agreed to take vitamins for six months. What they did not realize was that for half the time two of them would receive placebos. At the end of the first three months, those who had been given placebos were switched to the vitamins and vice versa. Each runner's performance increased dramatically for the three months he was taking the vitamins.

Vitamins are not drugs, but are nutrients required by every cell in your body. Since almost all foods are vitamin- and mineral-depleted, additional vitamins are essential for everyone. Supplements should always be taken daily, and not just occasionally. They are vital. Do not skip them. Do not think you are participating in a fad or joining the society of health nuts who swear by vitamins. You do yourself and your family and their offspring a grave disservice if you do not try to correct what generations of vitamin and mineral deficiency have done. You owe it to yourself and your great, great grandchildren. As the French physiologist Claude Bernard said, "All research starts on a bet, and ends on a bet; but you can hope that the result of your research is that you have improved your odds."[16]

Vitamins are co-enzymes that work in tandem with other nutrients and digestive enzymes to metabolize and utilize the food you eat. Vitamins do not replace food, they complement it. Once you begin to correct your vitamin and mineral imbalance, your body's natural immunity and healing processes will be armed to resist problems of aging and disease. Give your body what it needs to keep it operating on all its "cylinders."

NOTES

1. Michael Colgan, *Effects of Vitamin & Mineral Supplements on Physiology and Performance of Athletes and in Adjunctive Treatment of Certain Mental Disorders and Human Degenerative Diseases* (New Zealand: Colgan Institute of Nutritional Science), March 1981, p. 4. Dr. Colgan is a New Zealand scientist and visiting scholar at Rockefeller University in New York City.

2. "Contemporary Health Issues," Public Broadcasting System, Channel 10, Portland, OR: 10:30–11:00 AM, 13 February 1983.

3. Kathleen Stein, "Dr. C.'s Vitamin Elixers," *Omni*, April 1982, p. 70.

4. W. A. Price, *Nutrition and Physical Degeneration*, (Santa Monica: Price-Pottinger Nutrition Foundation, Heritage Edition, 1971; first published in 1937).

5. F. M. Pottinger, Jr., "The Effect of Heat Processed Foods and Metabolized Vitamin D Milk on the Dento-facial Structures of Experimental Animals," *American Journal of Orthodonture and Oral Surgery*, 32 (8) (1946): p. 467.

6. Marshall Mandell, M.D., and Lynne Waller Scanlon, *Dr. Mandell's 5-Day Allergy Relief System* (New York: T. Y. Crowell, 1979), p. 215.

7. Ibid., p. 216.

8. "Contemporary Health Issues."

9. Colgan, "Effects of Vitamin and Mineral Supplements," p. 2.

10. "Vitamins: The Key to Your Vitality," *Harpers Bazaar*, February 1982, p. 165.

11. "Contemporary Health Issues."

12. J. Marks, *Vitamins in Health and Disease* (London: J. and A. Churchill, 1968).

13. Colgan, "Effects of Vitamin and Mineral Supplements," p. 38.

14. Kathleen Stein, "Dr. C.'s Vitamin Elixers," *Omni*, April 1982, p. 70.

15. Guy E. Abraham, M.D., and Joel Hargrove, M.D., "Effect of Vitamin B-6 on Infertility in Women with Premenstrual Tension Syndrome" (Paper presented at the Thirty-fifth Annual Meeting of the American Fertility Society, San Francisco, Ca., February 5, 1979).

16. Dr. Jean Mayer, "This Much We Do Know," *Family Health*, Janaury 1981, p. 40.

13

Slim and Trim Forever?

FACT: You should never have to worry about dieting again after
The 21st Century Diet.

You Already Have What It Takes

Once you have completed the actual 21st Century Diet and
attained your desired weight, it is time to try your own wings. First
you have to gauge approximately how many calories per day you will
need to maintain your present weight by looking at the following
chart, "Approximate Calories Needed to Maintain Weight Levels."
This figure necessitates a little guesswork and "trial and error"
initially because you have to estimate the amount of calories burned
through physical activity, combine that information with knowledge
about your metabolism needs based on your age, height, and general
muscle-to-fat ratio, as well as acknowledge the impact of different
seasons on your instinctive ability to gain or lose weight. As mentioned earlier, age is an important factor because as you get older,
your hormone levels change and your ratio of muscle to fat shifts
away from muscle, making it more difficult to maintain muscle tone,
and your metabolic rate slows with each decade. Height is a crucial
factor when it comes to meeting basal or resting metabolism minimums.

The table on the following page is based on estimates by the
National Research Council. Use them only as a guide.

APPROXIMATE CALORIES NEEDED TO MAINTAIN WEIGHT LEVELS

FEMALE	AGE		
Weight	22	45	65
88	1,550	1,450	1,300
99	1,700	1,550	1,450
110	1,800	1,650	1,500
121	1,950	1,800	1,650
128	2,000	1,850	1,700
132	2,050	1,900	1,750
143	2,200	2,000	1,850
154	2,300	2,100	1,900
MALE			
110	2,200	2,000	1,850
121	2,350	2,150	1,950
132	2,500	2,300	2,100
143	2,650	2,400	2,200
154	2,800	2,600	2,400
165	2,950	2,700	2,500
176	3,050	2,800	2,600
187	3,200	2,950	2,700
198	3,350	3,100	2,800
209	3,500	3,200	2,900
220	3,700	3,400	3,100

The Food Families table in the Appendix includes caloric content as well as carbohydrate, protein, and fat levels. Concoct your own recipes following the rules of The 21st Century Diet. You know what it takes to maintain your new weight and your health:

• You must rotate your foods by not eating the same foods or foods from the same family too frequently.
• You must concentrate the majority (51 percent or more) of your higher calorie foods in meals that are eaten during the daytime.
• You must eat predominantly high protein meals during the daytime and predominantly high carbohydrate meals at night.

- You must be a member of a "moral support" group AND/OR maintain or increase physical activity at reasonable levels.
- You must take vitamin and mineral supplements.

Sorting Through Governmental and Institutional Dietary Recommendations

In 1977, there was a miniriot among the government hierarchy and lobbyists in Washington, D.C., when Senator George McGovern (D., South Dakota) released the results of a study undertaken by the Senate Select Committee on Nutrition to determine an ideal national nutrition policy. As chairman of the subcommittee, he issued six United States dietary goals that were very specific about ideal quantities of fat, carbohydrates, protein, and salt. One of the study's recommendations was to eat less meat as a protein source. So overwhelming and vociferous was the negative response by interested parties involved or connected with the meat industry that in 1980 a new report was issued by the Department of Agriculture and the Department of Health, Education, and Welfare (now the Department of Health and Human Services). Their twenty-page pamphlet called "Dietary Guidelines for Americans" was the culmination, according to Dan Greenberg, columnist and Washington observer, of "a long wait for little advice."[1] It did not offend anyone and it did not draw any counterfire. "Dietary Guidelines for Americans" made the following recommendations:

1. Add variety to your diet.
2. Maintain an ideal weight.
3. Avoid too much fat.
4. Eat foods containing sufficient starch and fiber.
5. Avoid sugar.
6. Avoid too much sodium.
7. Drink in moderation.

What about specifics? How much fat is too much fat? How do you know when you have had the proper amount of starch and fiber? Where do you draw the line in terms of quantities of sugar? Is too much salt two shakes of the salt shaker or three? What is your

particular definition of drinking in moderation? Based on the brou-
haha that resulted the last time a report got "too specific," the
committee appears to have opted to be as noncommittal as possible.
Therefore, the answers seem to be found only in the reports of other
organizations.

About the same time as the Senate Select Committee on Nutrition
released its controversial findings, the United Nations Food and
Agricultural Organization published its daily dietary recommendations:

UNITED NATIONS FOOD AND AGRICULTURAL ORGANIZATION MACRONUTRIENT RECOMMENDATIONS

ITEM	CALORIC CONTENT
Protein	10–15%
Fat	30–35%
Carbohydrate	50–60%

*Researchers feel that protein consumption is about twice what it ought to be,
and that typical American diets are far too saturated in fats, and that carbohydrates (fruits, vegetables) get short shrift. As you formulate your own 21st century
menus, keep in mind the above protein, fat, and carbohydrate recommendations.*

As a general admonishment, the recommendations included reduc-
tions in sugar and alcoholic beverages as well.[2] The American Heart
Association confirms the suggested amount of dietary fat recommended by the United Nations at approximately 30 percent (the
norm is 40 percent) and supports a limit of 300 milligrams of
cholesterol a day (the norm is 450 mg). There is some dispute about
the effect of cholesterol, however. Michael DeBakey, M.D., the
noted heart surgeon, feels that the problems associated with cholesterol are exaggerated. "A good 60 percent of the people who have
arteriosclerosis do not have elevated serum cholesterol levels," he
says.[3] Nonetheless, the thirty percent figure is a start.

The latest and ninth edition of the recommended daily dietary
allowances released by the National Academy of Sciences, Nutritional Research Council, Food and Nutrition Board (which has been

publishing about every five years since World War II), has suggested the following minimum for daily protein intake. Based on climate, economic status, and distribution of population, the recommendations are predicated on amounts high enough to maintain good nutrition in "healthy" persons in the United States. Bear in mind, however, that if you are less than perfectly healthy, your needs may differ, and that the recommendations do not take into account how much nutritional value is lost during the processing or preparation of food:

NATIONAL ACADEMY OF SCIENCE AND NUTRITIONAL RESEARCH COUNCIL RECOMMENDED DAILY DIETARY ALLOWANCES

| | | PROTEIN | | |
	Age	Height	Weight	Allowance
Males	19–51+	6'0"	154 pounds	56 grams
Females	19–51+	5'4"	120 pounds	44 grams

The average person consumes over 100 grams of protein each day, when all he or she really needs is about half that much (or the equivalent of one quarter-pound hamburger) for excellent health. If you are particularly active or tall, your protein requirement may increase slightly to reflect your increased metabolic needs, and you should adjust your protein intake accordingly. In general, however, man's daily protein consumption should remain within the 44 to 56 gram area.

The Reverse Pyramid Food Guide

In 1981, Jean A. T. Pennington of the Division of Nutrition, Food and Drug Administration, proposed a new food guide. Through an ever narrowing upside down pyramid, her guide visually defined and illustrated the relative contributions various food groups should make if you are to have a healthy diet. The reverse pyramid food guide takes into account the latest information about the inherent nutritional value of foods, and makes it quite apparent that the best diet is the diet "top heavy" with the foods that contain the most vitamins, minerals, and trace elements. To that end, note that this unique food guide emphasizes leafy vegetables, fruits, whole grains, refined grains, and legumes (in particular) as foods that should be eaten liberally. Low-fat milk, yogurt, and cheese, as well as lean meat, fish, and poultry should be eaten in moderation, while fatty and highly caloric foods such as whole milk and cheese, nuts, seeds, eggs, and fatty meats, game, and sausage should be eaten in limited quantities. Desserts, sweets, fats, and alcohol (with their empty calories and limited nutritional value) should barely be consumed at all—if at all!

As you formulate your own menus, keep the "reverse pyramid" in mind. Your daily diet should be heavy in leafy vegetables, fruits, legumes, whole grains, and refined grains. If you are going to use milk, try to make it skim or low fat to cut down on unnecessary amounts of fat. Keep your meat, fish, and poultry lean, cutting away the chucks of fat from your steak, choosing the less fatty fish, and

---

REVERSE PYRAMID FOOD GUIDE

Leafy vegetables, fruits, legumes (in particular), whole grains, and refined grains should dominate your diet, whereas desserts, sweets, fats, and alcoholic beverages should be extremely limited.

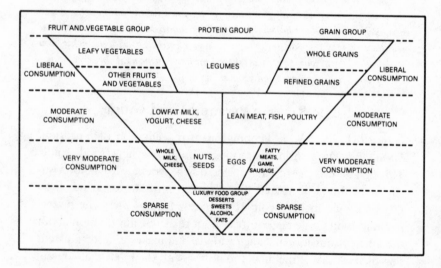

Source: "Considerations for a New Food Guide," *Journal of Nutrition Education*, vol. 13, no. 2, 1981. Copyright © Society of Nutrition Education.

trimming the skin from chicken. You will not only reduce calories, but you will reduce the amount of fat in your diet. When it comes to the luxury food groups, try to make eating rich desserts, slathering butter on your toast, and drinking milk shakes or alcoholic beverages a rarity. These items need not be *verboten,* but just a very limited part of your diet.

The 4-Day Food Rotation Guide

Throughout The 21st Century Diet you have been rotating your foods not only to increase the variety of foods you eat and to improve your overall health picture, but to help eliminate and prevent food allergies that have proved to result in the problem of food addiction. Mark Twain once said, "Habit is habit, and not to be flung out the window by any man, but coaxed downstairs a step at a time." The past weeks on The 21st Century Diet will have broken old habits. Continue the rotation process! Don't slip back into old habits.

The following list represents a suggested four-day rotation. It was created by taking many of the foods on the list in Chapter Three and only allowing a specific food *once* during the four-day rotation, and only allowing any other foods from that same "family" of foods to be eaten every other day, thus following the "rules" of food rotation. (These same choices, by the way, are the basis for the 800-, 1200-, and 1600-calorie menus in Chapter Ten. You may create your own rotation guide by taking the list in Chapter Three and dividing the families of foods up yourself. Some people create five-day, six-day, or seven-day rotations. It's up to you at this point. Just keep in mind that a four-day rotation should be the minimum rotation.) Glance at the various foods available from which to choose throughout the course of four days. Your selections each day should be checked for caloric and protein content against the Food Families List that follows in the Appendix. (A good book to use for additional reference, by the way, is *An Alternative Approach to Allergies* by Theron Randolph, M.D. Dr. Randolph is considered the premier researcher in the area of food allergies. His book goes into great detail about food rotation, etc.)

If a food is unfamiliar to you, do not reject it immediately. Give it a try. In particular, if you live in a culturally mixed neighborhood, chances are that enterprising groceries carry a little something for everyone. Ruffed grouse, rabbit, horsemeat, and rattlesnake may seem far-fetched to you, but these products are available . . . and often as close as a glance through the local telephone directory or a special order to your butcher. For more information, see Chapter Eleven, in which there appears a list of direct mail retailers and stores across the United States specializing in exotic foods or game. Fresh or frozen, they can get it to you by mail, or to your butcher.

DAY #1 FOOD CHOICES

Crab Family	crab
Flounder Family	dab, flounder, plaice
Hare Family	rabbit
Mackerel Family	skipjack, tuna
Pheasant Family	chicken, peafowl, pheasant, quail
Shrimp Family	shrimp

* * * *

Beech Family	chestnut
Cashew Family	cashew nut, mango, pistachio nut
Composite Family	artichoke, chicory, endive, escarole, Jerusalem artichoke, leaf lettuce, head lettuce
Gourd Family	cucumber, cantaloupe, casaba melon, crenshaw melon, honeydew melon, Persian melon, pumpkin
Lily Family	asparagus, chive, garlic clove, leek, onion, shallot
Miscellaneous Families	honey
Potato Family	tomato
Rose Family	apple, crabapple, pear
Sedge Family	Chinese water chestnut
Yam Family	yam

DAY #2 FOOD CHOICES

Bovine Family	beef (meat, butter, cheese, ice cream, milk, yogurt, veal), buffalo, goat (cheese, milk)
Red Snapper Family	red snapper
Swordfish Family	swordfish
Turkey Family	turkey

* * * *

Banana Family	banana, plantain
Buckwheat Family	buckwheat/kasha
Carrot Family	carrot, celery, parsley, parsnip
Fungi Family	mushroom
Grape Family	grape/raisin
Grass Family	rice (brown, white), rye, sugar cane, wheat germ, wild rice
Mustard Family	broccoli, Brussels sprouts, cabbage, cauliflower, celery cabbage, Chinese cabbage, collard greens, kale, kohlrabi, radish, rutabaga, turnip, watercress
Papaya Family	papaya
Rue Family	pomelo, tangelo, tangerine
Pineapple Family	pineapple
Walnut Family	black walnut, butternut, English walnut, hickory nut, pecan

DAY #3 FOOD CHOICES

Codfish Family	cod (scrod), cusk, haddock, pollack, tomcod
Deer Family	caribou, venison, elk, moose, reindeer
Lobster Family	crayfish, lobster
Mackerel Family	albacore, bonito, mackerel
Salmon Family	salmon species (Atlantic, coho, dog, king, pink, sockeye), trout species (brook, brown, lake, rainbow)
Sole Family	sole, turbot
Swine Family	hog (pork, bacon, ham, sausage, scrapple)

* * * *

Gourd Family	acorn squash, buttercup squash, butternut squash, caserta squash, cocozelle squash, crookneck squash, straightneck squash, cushaw squash, golden nugget squash, Hubbard squash, pattypan squash, turban squash, vegetable spaghetti squash, zucchini squash, watermelon
Heath Family	blueberry, cranberry
Laurel Family	avocado
Myrtle Family	guava
Potato Family	eggplant, green pepper, pepino, potato
Pedalium Family	sesame seed
Protea Family	macadamia nut
Rose Family	stone fruits (almond, apricot, cherry, nectarine, peach, plum/prune), berries (blackberry, black raspberry, boysenberry, dewberry, loganberry, purple raspberry, red raspberry, strawberry, youngberry)
Sapacaya Family	Brazil nut

DAY #4 FOOD CHOICES

Abalone Family	abalone
Bluefish Family	bluefish
Bovine Family	sheep (lamb, mutton)
Clam Family	clam, mussel
Duck Family	duck, goose
Halibut Family	halibut
Herring Family	Atlantic, Pacific, sardine, shad
Scallop Family	scallop

* * * *

Cactus Family	prickly pear
Goosefoot Family	beet, spinach
Grass Family	barley, corn, millet, oat
Honeysuckle Family	elderberry
Legume Family	alfalfa sprout, black-eyed pea, lentil, lima bean, mung sprout, navy bean, pea, peanut, soybean (tofu), string bean
Mallow Family	okra (gumbo)
Morning Glory Family	sweet potato
Mulberry Family	fig, mulberry
Olive Family	olive
Palm Family	coconut, date
Pomegranate Family	pomegranate
Rue Family	grapefruit, kumquat, orange
Saxifrage Family	gooseberry

Remember, there are more foods from which to choose; this is only a partial listing. Those foods that were not selected for this rotation plan may be added. You'll find them at the end of Chapter Ten under the heading "Substitute Foods."

Watch Out for Holiday Calories

If you have counted calories a thousand times, you'll be an old hand at the following list of food items. If you are new at calorie estimating, it may come as a surprise to you to discover that caloric content varies considerably from one food item to the next. A supper of chicken, peas, and carrots is truely "lean cuisine," as compared to a meal consisting of a steak, French fries, and salad laden with salad dressing. There is a reason that you gain weight when you eat a half a box of peanut cookies and wash them down with a quart of milk. And if you have never added up the potential caloric consumption over a holiday . . . be prepared for a shock. Even exercising restraint, you will discover that a Thanksgiving meal can range from as little as

THE CALORIE COUNTER'S THANKSGIVING

	CALORIES
2 slices whole wheat toast	140
2 tablespoons jam	100
1 cup raw vegetables	25
1/2 cup yogurt-based dip	60
1/4 pound steamed or boiled shrimp	100
1/2 cup cocktail sauce	120
10 crackers	110
1/2 pound white meat turkey, skinless	400
Baked potato with 1/2 teaspoon butter	170
1 cup mashed squash with butter	100
3/4 cup green beans with mushrooms	30
4 tablespoons defatted gravy	100
3/4 cup long grain and wild rice stuffing	225
1 cup tossed salad	30
5 tablespoons low-cal dressing	150
3 tablespoons cranberry sauce	75
1/8 of a mincemeat pie	320
3 tablespoons nondairy whipped topping	45
1 wine spritzer	50
Turkey sandwich snack	350
1/8 of pie snack	280
TOTAL	2,980

2,980 calories to 8,025 calories when you decide to throw caution to the winds!

Of course if you do not limit your caloric intake on the holidays and indulge yourself instead, it is entirely possible that you may consume enough calories to sustain you for four days or more, depending upon your size and activity levels. Take a look at the itemized list below. It represents a rather typical potential intake on Thanksgiving where the relatives arrive and the festivities begin in the early afternoon:

THE BINGER'S THANKSGIVING

6 pieces fudge	1,500
3 handfuls of nuts	800
2 alcoholic drinks	300
10 crackers with cheese	700
2 servings turkey	400
Mashed potatoes	200
Candied sweet potatoes	200
4 to 5 ladles gravy	1,000
3 tablespoons butter	300
1/2 cup sautéed green beans	150
2 cups squash, buttered	250
2 servings stuffing	600
Cranberry sauce	100
1 roll	100
2 pieces pie	800
3 cups coffee with cream, sugar	225
Stuffed celery	150
1 glass cider	150
TOTAL	8,025

Source: Patricia Weiss, "Have Another Helping—of Diet Advice," *USA Today,* 22 November 1982, p. 30. Adapted from Institute for Health Maintenance.

If you do binge on the holidays and on special occasions, be prepared to return to The 21st Century Diet for the next few days. Do not starve yourself as an overreaction to eating too much. Bear in mind that you do not want to mislead your body into thinking it is suddenly experiencing a famine. You want to avoid the instinctive metabolism change that makes it difficult to lose weight. The best approach, therefore, is to choose the appropriate 800-, 1200-, or 1600-calorie plan that is suitable for you *now*, based on your new weight and activity levels.

Watch Out for Subtle "Natural Changes" That Influence Weight Control

Keeping your weight under control entails being aware of the natural changes in your metabolism that slow it down or speed it up, or changes in your daily routine that alter your eating and/or activity levels. Pregnancy, the end of adolescence, retirement, a new job with *more* or *less* physical activity, a temporary or permanent injury, sickness, etc., are all capable of affecting your weight level. Don't be obsessive about your weight, but do monitor it occasionally by stepping on the scale periodically.

Begin or Keep Exercising

During the actual diet stage of The 21st Century Diet, you were given the option to exercise or not exercise. You still have that choice. However, if you opted to exercise as part of your diet program, keep it up . . . and expand your selection of activities. Diversify. Different exercises firm and tone different muscles. *Always keep the fun factor in mind, however, as the crucial ingredient to maintaining a sustained level of interest in any activity.*

If you chose not to exercise during the course of The 21st Century Diet, now that you have reached your ideal weight, consider beginning a program of light exercise to tighten up your body. According to a study at Cornell University's Division of Nutritional Sciences, the process of eating raises your metabolic rate. Exercise (particularly beginning within 45 minutes of your meal) increases metabolic rate even further, thus facilitating weight maintenance or weight loss. There is also mounting evidence that exercise lowers your "set-point"—the average weight you maintain without dieting—by, in a sense, turning up your metabolism's idling speed for more efficient weight control and caloric burning. Simply walking briskly is a fine initial exercise that anyone can undertake. If you know how to swim, dive in and start stroking and kicking your way to a better looking (and feeling) body. A study by Dr. Peter Wood of Stanford University Medical School also indicates that vigorous exercise at least once a day carries with it a momentum that affects the metabolism for up to 15 hours. Exercise twice a day and you will have metabolism that is accelerated 'round the clock.

Reread the suggested activities list in Chapter Eight. Now that you are slim, you may feel differently about joining in an activity that you avoided prior to weight loss. As always, keep the fun factor in mind, but give an activity a chance to grow in appeal. Try various choices for a week or two at least.

Eat "Close to Natural" Foods

In 1910, ten percent of food eaten by Americans was refined or treated with artificial additives. By 1981, eighty percent of the food on the American table was "processed" with colorings, additives, emulsifiers, preservatives, and the like. From 1940 to 1976, food coloring increased almost one hundred percent. In fact, the average American family eats nine pounds of additives annually. According to *Consumer Reports,* bread for your lunch sandwich contains additives to keep the bread fresh longer, the margarine has artificial coloring to make it look pale yellow, any salad dressing you might use contains emulsifiers to keep it from separating, and meat contains nitrates as a preservative. If you opt for soup along with lunch, every spoonful contains additives to combat rancidness. A cola drink is a chemical cocktail consisting of coloring, flavoring, sweetener, and artificial carbonation. Over 10,000 manmade chemical compounds are available to be added to your food supply. And this does not even take into account the "unintentional additives" that find their way to your plate in the form of pesticide residue, drugs that were administered or fed to livestock, and those chemicals that migrate from something as seemingly harmless as a plastic bag container.

In order to remedy the situation, you should get as close to natural foods as possible, preferably organically grown. If that is not practical, then do your best to select fresh, unadulterated vegetables and fruits. (Cucumbers and apples are notorious for having been lightly waxed to create or enhance a shine. Wax is a petroleum product, and you are not designed to eat wax.) Also, when you do cook, do a great deal of steaming of vegetables, rather than frying. The nutrients are better retained and no tars are formed.

The 21st Century Diet

If you had been living in Greece in 700 B.C. you would have lived to an average age of 18. In England in the sixteenth century you might have made it to 33. But in the 21st century you can expect to have to deal with your weight and health until an average age of 71.4 years if you are male and 78.7 years if you are female.[4] That is a lot of years to worry about your weight and constantly diet and rediet. The 21st Century Diet can make chronic dieting obsolete . . . and easy weight maintenance a pleasure.

The cartoon character Pogo once said, "Life is filled with insurmountable opportunities." The 21st Century Diet provides you with the chance to alter your approach to weight . . . and food . . . and motion. Once you get organized and approach weight maintenance as if it were as normal and natural a routine as brushing your teeth (you aren't obsessive about it, you just do it because you know you have to if you want to avoid cavities and have fresh breath), and you automatically do the right things; they become "second nature" to you. As you proceed from here, you should have no difficulty. Maintain the general rules and regulations of The 21st Century Diet. Maintain your support system. And maintain your ideal weight . . . forever.

NOTES

1. Daniel S. Greenberg, "A Long Wait for Little Advice," *Nutrition Today*, March/April 1980, pp. 20–22.

2. *Journal of Nutrition Education*, vol. 12, no. 2 (supplement 1980), p. 108.

3. Delma Heyn, "The Nutrition Free-for-All," *Family Health*, January 1981, pp. 24–25.

4. Mary Batten, "Life Spans," *Science Digest*, February 1984, p. 51.

APPENDIX

Food Families

3½-ounce servings or slightly less than one-half cup, unless otherwise stated

ANIMALS

	Calories	Protein (grams)	Fats (grams)	Carbohydrates (grams)
Amphibians				
Frog family				
bullfrog (4 legs)	73	16.4	.3	0

* * * *

	Calories	Protein (grams)	Fats (grams)	Carbohydrates (grams)
Birds				
Dove Family				
dove*	—	—	—	—
pigeon (squab)	142	17.5	7.5	0
Duck Family				
duck (skinless)				
domestic	165	16.0	8.2	0
wild	138	21.3	5.2	0
egg, 1	142	9.9	10.7	.5
goose	233	33.9	9.8	0
egg, 1	166	12.5	12.0	1.2
Grouse Family				
ruffed grouse (partridge)*	—	—	—	—
prairie chicken*	—	—	—	—
Guinea Fowl Family				
guinea fowl	158	23.4	6.4	0
eggs*	—	—	—	—
Pheasant Family				
chicken:				
light meat (skinless)	117	23.4	1.9	0
dark meat (skinless)	130	20.6	4.7	0
egg, 1	80	6.3	5.2	.4
Cornish hen*	—	—	—	—

*Information unavailable

Food Families

3½-ounce servings or slightly less than one-half cup, unless otherwise stated

ANIMALS

	Calories	Protein (grams)	Fats (grams)	Carbohydrates (grams)
peafowl*	—	—	—	—
pheasant	162	23.6	6.8	0
quail	172	25.4	7.0	0
egg, 1	16	1.3	1.1	trace
Turkey Family				
turkey	190	31.5	6.1	0
egg, 1	85	6.0	5.0	.8

* * * *

Crustaceans

	Calories	Protein (grams)	Fats (grams)	Carbohydrates (grams)
Crab Family				
crab	93	17.3	1.9	.5
Lobster Family				
crayfish	72	14.6	.5	1.2
lobster	91	16.9	1.9	.5
Shrimp Family				
prawn*	—	—	—	—
shrimp	91	18.1	.8	1.5

* * * *

Fish (freshwater)

	Calories	Protein (grams)	Fats (grams)	Carbohydrates (grams)
Catfish Family				
catfish	103	17.6	3.1	0
yellow bullheads	103	17.6	3.1	0
Eel Family				
eel	233	15.9	18.3	0
Herring Family				
roe, shad	130	42.4	2.3	1.5
Minnow Family				
carp	115	18.0	4.2	0
chub	145	15.3	8.8	0
Muskellunge Family				
Northern pike	88	18.3	0.0	0
pickerel	84	18.7	.5	0

*Information unavailable

Food Families

3½-ounce servings or slightly less than one-half cup, unless otherwise stated

ANIMALS

	Calories	Protein (grams)	Fats (grams)	Carbohydrates (grams)
Paddlefish Family				
North American				
paddlefish*	—	—	—	—
Perch Family				
perch, yellow	91	19.5	.9	0
pike	84	18.7	.5	0
sauger	84	17.9	.8	0
walleye	93	19.3	1.2	0
Salmon Family				
salmon species:				
Atlantic	217	22.5	13.4	0
coho	153	20.8	7.1	0
dog	156	17.6	9.0	0
king	105	18.3	3.0	0
pink	119	20.0	3.8	0
sockeye	171	20.3	9.3	0
trout species:				
brook	101	19.2	2.1	0
brown*	—	—	—	—
lake	168	18.3	10.3	0
rainbow	195	21.5	11.4	0
Smelt Family				
smelt	98	18.6	2.1	0
Sturgeon Family				
beluga*	—	—	—	—
sturgeon caviar				
(granular)	262	26.9	15.0	3.3
Sucker Family				
bigmouth buffalofish	113	17.5	4.2	0
black buffalofish	113	17.5	4.2	0
sucker	104	20.6	1.8	0
Sunfish Family				
black bass species:	93	19.2	1.2	0
largemouth	—	—	—	—

*Information unavailable

Food Families

3½-ounce servings or slightly less than one-half cup, unless otherwise stated

ANIMALS

	Calories	Protein (grams)	Fats (grams)	Carbohydrates (grams)
smallmouth	—	—	—	—
spotted	—	—	—	—
bluegill*	—	—	—	—
sunfish species:				
longear sunfish*	—	—	—	—
pumpkinseed*	—	—	—	—
crappie	79	14.6	.5	1.2
Whitefish Family				
lake whitefish	155	18.9	8.2	0

Fish (saltwater)

	Calories	Protein (grams)	Fats (grams)	Carbohydrates (grams)
Anchovy Family				
anchovy	176	19.2	10.3	0
Barracuda Family				
barracuda	113	21.0	2.6	0
Bluefish Family				
bluefish	117	20.5	3.3	0
Codfish Family				
cod (scrod)	78	17.6	.3	0
cusk	75	17.2	.2	0
haddock	165	19.6	6.4	0
pollack	95	20.4	.9	0
tomcod	77	17.2	.4	0
Conger Eel Family				
conger eel*	—	—	—	—
Croaker Family				
croaker	96	17.8	2.2	0
drum, red	80	18.0	.4	0
sea trout	195	21.5	11.4	0
silver perch*	—	—	—	—
spot	219	17.6	15.9	0
weakfish	121	16.5	5.6	0
Flounder Family				
dab	79	16.7	.8	0

*Information unavailable

Food Families

3½-ounce servings or slightly less than one-half cup, unless otherwise stated

ANIMALS

	Calories	Protein (grams)	Fats (grams)	Carbohydrates (grams)
flounder	79	16.7	.8	0
plaice	79	16.7	.8	0
Grunt Family				
gray*	—	—	—	—
common*	—	—	—	—
yellow*	—	—	—	—
Gurnard Family				
sea robin*	—	—	—	—
sea tag*	—	—	—	—
Halibut Family				
halibut	100	20.9	1.2	0
Harvestfish Family				
butterfish	169	18.1	10.2	0
harvestfish	95	16.2	2.9	0
Herring Family				
Atlantic	176	17.3	11.3	0
Pacific	98	17.5	2.6	0
sardine	160	19.2	8.6	0
shad	170	18.6	10.0	0
Jack Family				
amberjack*	—	—	—	—
jack mackerel	143	21.6	5.6	0
pompano	166	18.8	9.5	0
yellow jack*	—	—	—	—
Mackerel Family				
albacore	177	25.3	7.6	0
bonito	168	24.0	7.3	0
mackerel	191	19.0	12.2	0
skipjack	143	21.6	5.6	0
tuna	145	25.2	4.1	0
Marlin Family				
marlin*	—	—	—	—
sailfish*	—	—	—	—

*Information unavailable

Food Families

3½-ounce servings or slightly less than one-half cup, unless otherwise stated

ANIMALS

	Calories	Protein (grams)	Fats (grams)	Carbohydrates (grams)
Porgy Family				
scup (porgy)	112	19.0	3.4	0
Puffer Family				
puffer*	—	—	—	—
Red Snapper Family				
red snapper	93	19.8	0.9	0
Sea Bass Family				
bass, yellow	88	18.0	2.3	0
grouper	87	19.3	.5	0
perch, white	91	19.3	4.0	0
sea bass	96	21.4	.5	0
Sea Catfish Family				
ocean catfish*	—	—	—	—
Scorpionfish Family				
rosefish (ocean perch)	88	18.0	1.2	0
Shark Family				
shark	—	—	—	—
Silverside Family				
mullet	146	19.6	6.9	0
silverside*	—	—	—	—
whitebait*	—	—	—	—
Sole Family				
sole	79	16.7	8.0	0
turbot*	—	—	—	—
Swordfish Family				
swordfish	118	19.2	4.0	0
Tarpon Family				
tarpon*	—	—	—	—
Tilefish Family				
tilefish	79	17.5	.5	0

*Information unavailable

Food Families

3½-ounce servings or slightly less than one-half cup, unless otherwise stated

ANIMALS

	Calories	Protein (grams)	Fats (grams)	Carbohydrates (grams)
Mammals				
Bear Family				
bear*	—	—	—	—
Beaver Family				
beaver	248	29.2	0.0	0
Bovine Family				
beef cattle				
beef:				
lean and fat	286	27.0	19.0	0
lean only	196	31.0	7.0	0
butter	716	.6	81.0	.4
cheese	See Appendix for list of various cheeses.			
ice cream	207	4.0	12.5	20.6
milk:				
whole, 1 cup	149	8.0	8.1	11.4
low fat, 1 cup	122	8.1	4.7	11.7
oleomargarine	720	.6	81.0	.4
yogurt:				
low fat	143	11.9	3.4	16.0
whole	141	7.9	7.7	10.4
veal	173	19.4	10.0	0
buffalo*	—	—	—	—
goat (kid):	165	18.7	0.0	0
cheese*	—	—	—	—
goat's milk	67	3.2	4.0	4.6
sheep:				
lamb:				
chop, 1 lean	103	12.5	.9	0.0
leg, 1 slice	96	13.8	.6	0.0
mutton (mature sheep)*	—	—	—	—

*Information unavailable

Food Families

3½-ounce servings or slightly less than one-half cup, unless otherwise stated

ANIMALS

	Calories	Protein (grams)	Fats (grams)	Carbohydrates (grams)
Deer Family				
caribou, lean	127	21.8	3.8	0
elk*	—	—	—	—
moose*	—	—	—	—
reindeer	127	21.8	3.8	0
venison	126	21.0	4.0	0
Hare Family				
rabbit:				
domestic	162	21.0	8.0	0
wild	135	21.0	5.0	0
Horse Family				
horse	118	18.1	0.0	0
Opposum Family				
opposum	221	30.2	10.2	0
Pronghorn Family				
antelope*	—	—	—	—
Squirrel Family				
prairie dog*	—	—	—	—
squirrel*	—	—	—	—
woodchuck*	—	—	—	—
Swine Family				
hog:				
bacon, 2 slices	86	5.0	8.0	.1
ham	193	18.3	12.3	.9
pork, canned	193	18.3	12.3	.9
sausage, 1 link	94	3.5	8.8	0.0
scrapple, 3½ ounces	215	8.8	13.6	14.6
Whale Family				
whale	156	20.6	7.5	0

* * * *

Mollusks

	Calories	Protein (grams)	Fats (grams)	Carbohydrates (grams)
Abalone Family				
abalone	98	18.7	.5	3.4

*Information unavailable

Food Families

3½-ounce servings or slightly less than one-half cup, unless otherwise stated

ANIMALS

	Calories	Protein (grams)	Fats (grams)	Carbohydrates (grams)
Clam Family				
clam (4 large)	82	14.0	1.9	1.3
mussel, meat	95	14.4	2.2	3.3
Octopus Family				
octopus	73	15.3	.8	0
Oyster Family				
oyster (8 medium):				
eastern	66	8.4	1.8	3.4
western	97	10.6	2.2	6.4
Scallop Family				
bay scallop	81	15.3	.2	3.3
sea scallop	81	15.3	.2	3.3
Snail Family				
snail	90	16.1	1.4	2.0
Squid Family				
squid	84	16.4	.9	1.5

* * * *

Reptiles

	Calories	Protein (grams)	Fats (grams)	Carbohydrates (grams)
Snapping Turtle Family				
snapping turtle*	—	—	—	—
Diamondback Terrapin Family				
diamondback terrapin	111	18.6	0.0	0
green turtle	89	19.8	.5	0
eggs, 3 to 5	115	12.6	6.3	0
Rattler Family				
diamondback rattlesnake*	—	—	—	—

*Information unavailable

Food Families

3½ ounce servings or slightly less than one-half cup, unless otherwise stated

PLANTS

	Calories	Protein (grams)	Fats (grams)	Carbohydrates (grams)
Banana Family				
banana	85	1.1	.2	22.2
plantain	119	1.1	.4	31.2
Beech Family				
chestnut:				
dried (1 cup)	377	6.7	4.1	78.6
fresh (6)	194	2.9	1.5	42.1
Birch Family				
filbert (hazelnut) (12)	97	1.6	9.5	3.0
Buckwheat Family				
buckwheat:				
whole grain				
(1 cup, raw)	335	11.6	2.4	72.9
Cactus Family				
prickly pear	42	.5	.1	10.9
Carpetweed Family				
New Zealand spinach	19	2.2	.3	3.1
Carrot Family				
carrot	42	1.1	.2	9.7
celery	17	.9	.1	3.9
parsley	44	3.6	.6	8.5
parsnip	76	1.7	.5	17.5
Cashew Family				
cashew nuts (8)	84	2.0	6.9	4.4
mango	66	.7	.4	16.8
pistachio nuts (30)	88	2.9	8.0	2.8
Composite Family				
artichoke	44	2.9	.2	10.6
chicory	20	1.8	.3	3.8
endive	20	1.7	.1	4.1
escarole	20	1.7	.1	4.1
Jerusalem artichoke	44	2.9	.2	10.6

Food Families

3½ ounce servings or slightly less than one-half cup, unless otherwise stated

PLANTS

	Calories	Protein (grams)	Fats (grams)	Carbohydrates (grams)
lettuce:				
head	13	.9	.1	2.9
leaf	18	1.3	.3	3.5
Fungi Family				
mushrooms	28	2.7	.3	4.4
Goosefoot Family				
beet	43	1.6	.1	9.9
spinach, cooked	22	2.4	0.0	3.2
Gourd Family				
cucumber	15	.9	.1	3.4
muskmelon:				
cantaloupe	30	.7	.1	7.5
casaba	27	1.2	trace	6.5
crenshaw	30	.7	.1	7.5
honeydew	33	.8	.3	7.7
Persian	30	.7	.1	7.5
pumpkin	26	1.0	.1	6.5
squash:				
acorn	44	1.5	.1	11.2
buttercup	54	1.4	.1	.1
butternut	54	1.4	.1	.1
caserta	44	1.5	.1	11.2
cocozelle	17	1.2	.1	3.6
crookneck	20	1.2	.2	4.3
cushaw	20	1.2	.2	4.3
golden nugget	20	1.2	.2	4.3
Hubbard	39	1.4	.3	9.4
pattypan	20	1.2	.2	4.3
straightneck	20	1.2	.2	4.3
turban	20	1.2	.2	4.3
vegetable spaghetti*	—	—	—	—
zucchini	17	1.2	.8	3.6

*Information unavailable

Food Families

3½ ounce servings or slightly less than one-half cup, unless otherwise stated

PLANTS

	Calories	Protein (grams)	Fats (grams)	Carbohydrates (grams)
watermelon	20	1.2	.2	4.3
Grass Family				
barley, pearled				
(½ cup)	349	8.2	1.0	78.8
corn, sweet (1 ear)	96	3.5	1.0	22.1
millet, whole grain	327	9.9	2.9	72.9
oats, meal,				
(1 cup cooked)	148	5.4	2.8	26.0
rice:				
brown (½ cup cooked)	89	1.9	.5	19.1
puffed cereal (1 cup)	54	.9	0.0	12.6
white (½ cup cooked)	82	1.5	.1	18.1
rye, bread (1 slice)	56	2.1	.3	12.0
sugarcane (1 teaspoon)	16	2.1	0.0	4.0
wheat germ (1 tablespoon)	36	2.7	1.1	4.7
wild rice (¼ cup raw)	99	3.9	.2	21.1
Grape Family				
grapes (22):	69	1.3	1.0	15.7
raisins (½ cup)	289	2.5	.2	77.4
Heath Family				
blueberry	62	.7	.5	15.3
cranberry	46	.4	.7	10.8
Honeysuckle Family				
elderberry	72	2.6	.5	16.4
Laurel Family				
avocado, ½	167	2.1	16.4	6.3
Legume Family				
alfalfa sprouts (2 ounces)	20	2.0	0.0	2.0

Food Families

3½ ounce servings or slightly less than one-half cup, unless otherwise stated

PLANTS

	Calories	Protein (grams)	Fats (grams)	Carbohydrates (grams)
black-eyed peas, dried (½ cup)	130	.4	9.0	22.1
lentils (⅔ cup cooked)	106	7.8	trace	19.3
limas	123	8.4	.5	22.1
mung sprouts (1⅔ cups)	35	3.8	.2	6.6
navy bean*	—	—	—	—
peas	84	6.3	.4	14.4
peanuts:	564	26.0	47.5	18.6
peanut butter (3 tablespoons)	288	13.0	23.9	10.5
soybeans:				
curd (tofu), 3½ ounces	72	7.8	4.2	2.4
dried	403	34.1	17.7	33.5
string bean	32	1.9	.2	7.1
Lily Family				
asparagus (6 stalks)	26	2.5	.2	5.0
chives (1 tablespoon)	3	.2	0.0	.1
garlic clove (1)	4	.2	0.0	0
leeks (4)	52	2.2	.3	11.2
onion (1 tablespoon)	4	.2	trace	.9
shallot (1¾ ounces)	72	2.5	.1	16.8
Mallow Family				
okra/gumbo (9 pods)	36	2.4	.3	7.6
Miscellaneous Family				
honey (1 tablespoon)	61	.1	0.0	16.5
Morning Glory Family				
sweet potato	114	1.7	4.0	26.3
Mulberry Family				
fig, 2 large	80	1.2	.3	20.3
mulberries (¾ cup)	62	1.2	0.0	14.6

*Information unavailable

Food Families

3½ ounce servings or slightly less than one-half cup, unless otherwise stated

PLANTS

	Calories	Protein (grams)	Fats (grams)	Carbohydrates (grams)
Mustard Family				
broccoli	32	3.6	.3	5.9
Brussels sprouts	45	4.9	.4	8.3
cabbage	24	1.3	.2	5.4
cauliflower	27	2.7	.2	5.2
celery cabbage	14	1.2	.1	3.0
Chinese cabbage	14	1.2	.1	3.0
collard greens	45	4.8	.8	7.5
kale	53	6.0	.8	9.0
kohlrabi	29	2.0	.1	6.6
radishes	17	1.0	.1	3.6
rutabaga	46	1.1	.1	11.0
turnip	30	1.0	.2	6.6
watercress	19	2.2	.3	3.0
Myrtle Family				
guava	62	.8	.6	15.0
Olive Family				
olive, green (2)	30	.4	1.6	.2
olive, ripe (2)	37	.2	4.0	.6
Palm Family				
coconut:				
dried (2 tablespoons)	83	.5	.3	8.0
fresh (½ cup)	174	1.2	17.6	4.7
date (10 medium)	274	2.2	.5	72.9
Papaya Family				
papaya	39	.6	.1	10.0
Pedalium Family				
sesame seeds, dried	563	18.6	49.1	21.6
Pineapple Family				
pineapple	52	.4	.2	13.7
Pomegranate Family				
pomegranate, pulp	63	.5	.3	16.4

Food Families

3½ ounce servings or slightly less than one-half cup, unless otherwise stated

PLANTS

	Calories	Protein (grams)	Fats (grams)	Carbohydrates (grams)
Potato Family				
eggplant	25	1.2	2.0	5.6
green pepper	22	1.2	.2	4.8
pepino*	—	—	—	—
potato	76	2.1	.1	17.1
tomato	22	1.1	2.0	4.7
Protea Family				
macadamia nuts (6)	109	1.4	11.7	1.5
Rose Family				
pomes:				
apple	58	.2	.6	14.5
crabapple	68	.4	.3	17.8
pear	61	.7	.4	15.3
stone fruits:				
almonds, dried	598	18.6	54.2	19.5
apricot	51	1.0	.2	12.8
cherry:				
sour	58	1.2	.3	14.3
sweet	70	1.3	.3	17.4
nectarine	64	.6	trace	17.1
peach	38	.6	.1	9.7
plum or prune	66	.5	trace	17.8
berries:				
blackberries	58	1.2	.9	12.9
black raspberries	73	1.5	1.4	15.7
boysenberries	58	1.2	.9	12.9
dewberries	58	1.2	.9	12.9
loganberries	62	1.0	.6	14.9
loneberries*	—	—	—	—
purple raspberries*	—	—	—	—
raspberries	73	1.5	1.4	15.7
red raspberries	73	1.5	1.4	15.7
strawberries	37	.7	.5	8.4

*Information unavailable

Food Families

3½ ounce servings or slightly less than one-half cup, unless otherwise stated

PLANTS

	Calories	Protein (grams)	Fats (grams)	Carbohydrates (grams)
youngberries	58	1.2	.9	12.9
Rue (Citrus) Family				
grapefruit, ½	41	.5	.1	10.6
kumquat, 6	65	.9	.1	17.1
orange, 1	49	1.0	.2	12.2
pomelo*	—	—	—	—
tangelo, 1	41	.5	.1	9.7
tangerine, 1	43	.5	.2	10.1
Sapacaya Family				
Brazil nuts (4)	97	2.2	2.8	1.7
Saxifrage Family				
gooseberries	39	.8	.2	9.7
Sedge Family				
water chestnuts (Chinese) (8)	40	.8	0.0	9.8
Spurge Family				
tapioca, dry (1 tablespoon)	35	trace	0.0	8.1
Walnut Family				
black walnut (4)	94	2.7	8.7	2.8
butternut (5)	96	3.6	9.2	1.3
English walnut (1 tablespoon, chopped)	49	1.1	4.8	1.2
hickorynut (15)	101	2.1	10.1	2.0
pecan (6)	104	1.4	11.0	2.0
Yam Family				
Yam:				
American*	—	—	—	—
Chinese	101	2.1	.2	23.2

*Information unavailable

Protein and Caloric Content of Cheeses

Although cheese is one of those products that is usually eaten in bite-sized pieces, each piece often contains a great many calories. One ounce of cheese (about the size of a large sugar cube!) can add 100 calories with each slice of the cheese cutter. Therefore, cheese intake has to be monitored carefully. Take a look at the list below:

CHEESE 1 Ounce

TYPE	PROTEIN	CALORIES
American	6.5 grams	107
Blue	6.0	103
Brick	6.2	103
Brie	5.8	94
Camembert	4.9	84
Caraway	7.0	105
Cheddar	7.0	112
Cheezola	7.0	89
Cheshire	6.5	108
Colby	6.7	110
Cottage, 1 cup		
creamed	30.5	239
uncreamed, 1% fat	28.0	163
uncreamed, 2% fat	31.1	203
Cream cheese	2.1	99
Edam	7.7	87
Feta	4.0	74
Fontina	7.2	109
Gjetost	2.7	130
Gouda	7.0	100
Gruyere	8.1	115
Liederkranz	4.6	85
Limburger	5.7	93
Lite-Line	7.3	52
Monterey	6.8	105
Mozzarella	5.4	79
Muenster	6.6	104

CHEESE 1 Ounce *(cont'd.)*

TYPE	PROTEIN	CALORIES
Neufchatel	2.8	73
Parmesan	10.1	111
Port du Salut	6.7	99
Provolone	7.4	98
Ricotta, 1/2 cup	14.5	216
Romano	9.0	110
Roquefort	6.1	105
Swiss	7.7	106
Tilsit	6.8	95

Fruit and Vegetable Drink Calories

The following is a list of fruit and vegetable juices that are commonly available either as frozen concentrates (to be diluted with water later) or as extracts contained in bottles or cans. Bear in mind if you want to drink a food instead of eat it, that you should read labels carefully to make certain that there is no sugar added to your selection.

FRUIT AND VEGETABLE DRINKS
Approximately ½ Cup

JUICE	CALORIES
apple	58
apricot	61
blackberry	46
blueberry	67
carrot	48
cranberry	32
currant, black	69
grape	82
grapefruit	49
guava	86
loganberry	50
orange	56
papaya	60
peach	59
pear	64
pineapple	69
prune	92
raspberry	49
tangelo	51
tangerine	53
tomato	22

INDEX

Longevity, ideal weight and, 45–46
Lunch
  calorie consumption at, 42
  protein needs at, 2, 33, 35–37, 147–48, 172
  See also Plans and Menus, 21st Century Diet

McGovern, George, 173
Magnesium, 167
Mail-order sources for exotic foods, 149–50
Malnutrition, 131
  studies, 158–60, 168
Mandell, Marshall, xv
Marriage, weight gain and, 67–68
Measuring foods, 147
Meat consumption, excessive, 9–11
  See also Animal protein; Protein
Meat-eating instinct, 2, 9–10
Medication, fasting and, 86
Megavitamin therapy, for mental problems, 160–61
Mental problems
  food addiction and, 72
  vitamin deficiency and, 160–61
Menus, *see* Plans and Menus, 21st Century Diet; Recipes
Metabolic rate, 4–5
  changes, 34–35, 62–63
  exercise and, 93–94, 98
  famine instinct and, 68–70, 86
  minimum caloric intake and, 5, 131–32
  rebound weight gain and, 68–70
Methylated xanthines, 38–39
  in beverages and drugs (charts), 40, 41
  See also Caffeine
Metropolitan Life Insurance Company height/weight chart, 46–47
Migraine headaches, 72, 146

Mineral supplements, *see* Supplements, vitamin and mineral
Moral support group, 94–95, 101–2, 106–7, 173
Motivation for weight loss
  enjoyment as key, 91–93, 102
  personal goals as, 90–91
Mouthwash, 87
Muscle-to-fat ratios, 47–50
  aging and, 63
  ideal weights for men and women and (charts), 49
  measuring, 48
  See also Exercise

National Academy of Sciences and Nutritional Research Council recommended daily intakes
  of protein, 174–75
  of salt, 145
National Institute on Aging, 45
"Natural" food sources, 161–62, 165
  deficiencies in, 3, 161–64, 168–69
Niacin, 160–61
Nursing women, weight gain and, 64

Obese Patient, The (Bray), 68–69
Obesity, extreme, 117–18
  plan and menus for, 116–23
  See also Food addiction
Obesity Research Clinic (New York), 63
Omnivores, 16
Organic soil, 165
Optional Athletic Activities (checklist), 96–97
Overcoming Jet Lag (Ehret and Scanlon), xvi